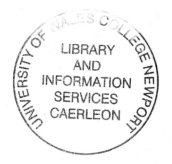

Transforming Community Care: a distorted vision?

Helen Gorman and Karen Postle

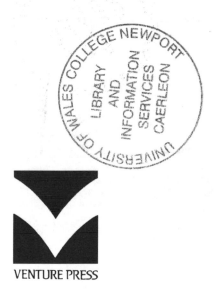

VENTURE PRESS

BASW website: http://www.basw.co.uk

Published by
VENTURE PRESS
16 Kent Street
Birmingham
B5 6RD

British Library Cataloguing-in-Publication Data
A catalogue record for this book is available from the British Library

ISBN   1 86178 059 1   (paperback)

Cover design by:
Western Arts
21b Highgate Close
London
N6 4SD

Printed in Great Britain by Hobbs the Printers Ltd, Totton, Hampshire

This book is dedicated to the memory of David Brandon (1941–2001). As editor of this book at its inception and throughout its writing we found him generous with time, ideas and encouragement. He will be remembered as someone who was a nagging conscience whenever and wherever social work is complacent, misguided or negligent. Sadly, David's illness and untimely death prevented him seeing this book to publication, but we hope we have done justice to his memory.

Contents   Page

Acknowledgements   v

1: Introduction   **1**
The state of the art: community care as entertainment?   1
The meaning of 'community' and the
      concept of community care   3
Community care as care management   7
Why this book, and who are these authors?   8
What the books aims to do   10
Outline of the book   10
Suggested background reading   12

2: Origins and Influences   **13**
The development of care management   13
Is care management a distortion of community care?   14
From new managerialism to best value   16
From professional social worker to the
      occupation of care manager?   20
The search for quality and the realities of audit   24
The mantra of partnership – is it working?   25
Conclusion   26

3: Any care or any management?   **29**
Introduction: a letter to the editor   29
Social worker to care manager – a changed role?   30
Care management – any care?   34

4: Decision making about community care services –
dithering as an art form?   **43**
Working inter-professionally: does it lead to better
      decisions for service users?   45
Decision-making in care management: does it matter
      who your care manager is?   48
Decision-making and acting as the
      'Street Level Bureaucrats' – a powerful
      role for care managers?   49
Accountability and the decision-making process   53
Decision-making and the community?   58
Conclusion: decision-making and community
      care in transition   59

5: Empowerment   **61**
  An overworked word or a meaningful concept?   61
  Notions of empowerment in care management   63
  Care management: empowering older people or
     exacerbating dependency?   65
  Care managers' responses to their work: coping with its
     ambiguities and tensions   69
  Implications of demoralised workers doing demoralising
     work in times of uncertainty and ambiguity   72
  Suggestions for further reading about empowerment   75

6. Conclusion   **77**
  An overview   77
  Implications for the future: deconstucting and reconstructing
     social work   81
  Community care in transition – towards learning organisations
     in health and social care?   85

Bibliography   **91**

Acknowledgements

Several people have seen this book through from the germ of an idea to its fruition, and we want to thank them. The suggestion for the book came from Malcolm Payne, and we thank him for that encouragement. The book is based on work from our doctoral theses; our research could not have taken place without the help and co-operation of social services staff. Although confidentiality prevents us from naming people or locations, we express our gratitude to those often hard-pressed staff who gave up time to take part in our research. Thanks are also due to our Ph.D. supervisors, Les Franklin, Gail Wilson, Paul Waddington, Graham Tuson and Joan Orme for their support and guidance.

From the time of David Brandon's illness, Toby Brandon offered invaluable help in reading drafts and making suggestions, and liaised with Shula Ramon who took on the editorial function. At a difficult time, when they had lost a father and friend, we have hugely valued their help and advice. Christine Sedgwick at Venture Press has been extremely patient and helpful with our questions.

Our colleagues at The University of Central England, Birmingham, and University College Chichester have supported us in this project, and our students have provided a constant reminder of the realities of care management.

Mick Gorman and Tony Postle have given support, encouragement and grammatical advice, and tolerated our dedication to this task just when they thought we'd surfaced from the rigours of doctoral study.

The mistakes, errors and omissions are all ours!

Chapter 1
Introduction

This book aims to explore what has become of the rhetoric of community care and how it has been translated, or possibly distorted, into various realities with particular reference to the impact of this translation for older people. A fuller introduction to our subject will be given later in this chapter, but we begin with an illustration of the reality of community care for one older person, a discussion of what can be understood by 'community' and a brief outline of the background to the NHS (National Health Service) and Community Care Act 1990.

The state of the art: community care as entertainment?
On 3 May 2001, BBC1 screened a 'Life of Grime Special' about Mr Trebus. This was the trailer in the *Radio Times*:

> *This update* [of a programme screened two years before] *has all the qualities that made the Polish war veteran's battle so fascinating: his anti-authoritarianism, his terrier-like refusal to see reason and his ability to live in squalor without apparently noticing.* (Lass, 2001, p 104)

To the accompaniment of lively music and a voice-over by an apparently bemused John Peel, the programme showed Mr Trebus's continuing conflict with his Local Authority's environmental health department. He hoarded rubbish to the point where this became a health hazard for both himself and his neighbours, and resisted all attempts to clear this or have repairs made to his property. One humane and kind local person, a retired businessman, decided to champion Mr Trebus's cause and help him in his battles with the authorities but gradually became worn down and frustrated by his attempts. As the trailer concluded:

> *After causing an immense amount of aggravation, he [Mr Trebus] turns to the camera with a face in which butter would refuse to melt to say: 'Have I done something wrong?'* (Lass, 2001 p 104)

Aside from wondering what constitutes entertainment and where our boundaries of public/private life lie, what does this programme tell us about how people are cared for within their communities today? Where were the professionals, such as a GP, social worker or district nurse? Perhaps they were 'unable to comment', leaving it to environmental health officers and the police to steal the limelight. Perhaps attempts to portray a more balanced view would not have made good television. Viewers saw an elderly man, a survivor of wartime atrocities, living away from his homeland, now reduced to a figure to be belittled and cajoled like a naughty child. While the sundry officials and the helpful businessman spoke of their admiration for his spirit, they all colluded in a display of 'entertainment' which would not have been out of place in nineteenth-century Bedlam!

Most social workers who have worked with older people have met someone very like Mr Trebus. In such situations there are always issues to explore, such as:

- How can I find out what makes this person tick? Who is he? What is his story? How has this come to be?
- What are the person's expressed wishes and how far do these conflict with risk to themselves or others?
- How great are those risks and how could they be managed?
- How much insight does the person have into their situation? How far are they able to make or participate in decisions about what should happen to them?
- Who else is in their support network? In Mr Trebus's case we never discovered what had become of his family and whether or not he was estranged from them. Similarly, we did not know if he had links with other members of the Polish community.
- How could informal networks be maximised and supported? The businessman who was supporting Mr Trebus was doing a fantastic job but feeling at an understandable loss about what to do next. He had apparently no source of support or (if he'd wanted it) advice/information.
- What is the medical opinion? All we were told was that Mr Trebus was 'not mentally ill' but, for example, at no point was the possibility of Diogenes syndrome (one of the most common reasons for hoarding apparently worthless objects) mentioned or investigated. He looked very frail but we had no information about his physical health

Social work is just one way of dealing with social problems, and many, if not most, people would prefer to resolve the problems in their lives without outside intervention. There are, however, situations in which the art of skilled social work intervention can make a difference, and we would suggest that Mr Trebus's situation could have been one of those.

Perhaps a social worker had worked with Mr Trebus over a long period of time but been unable to make any headway. Maybe, more worryingly, no one thought it worth contacting Social Services because it was known that Mr Trebus didn't fit neatly into quite the right category for their help. Perhaps there was an ongoing discussion across social work teams about whether he should have a social worker from the mental health team, the care of older people team, the community development team, or any other number of fragmented specialisations. Possibly a social worker had carried out a hasty risk assessment, informed Mr Trebus of her/his decision for action and closed his case when Mr Trebus had refused further help (as he surely would have done).

Whatever the reasons, the outcome was that, in 2001, we witnessed a proud, vulnerable person locked into a hopeless battle with innumerable authority figures in a situation which looked increasingly likely to result in his permanent removal from his home. This seems a very long way from what was intended by 'care in the community'.

The meaning of 'community' and the concept of community care

The story of Mr Trebus serves as an illustration of the difficulties inherent in trying to define what we mean by *community*, a necessary starting point for any book exploring the nature of community care. What could *community* have meant to Mr Trebus?

- A geographical location: the area where he lived with its mixture of housing, its long-term residents and people recently moved to the area.
- A supportive network of people who might be able to look out for one another's interests.
- A community of interest/similarity: people who shared some or much of his history as a Polish immigrant. Here we need to bear in mind the dangers of assumptions of homogeneity about any group of immigrant people, particularly from a country whose older population was divided by its wartime experience.
- A group united in its focus in a time of stress or difficulty. Sadly, Mr Trebus would be more likely to have been the unwelcome focus of this 'community'.
- A combination of parts of these or, perhaps most likely, none of them.

What we can conclude about our exploration of what, if anything, community might have meant for Mr Trebus is that this is a very debatable term (Bornat, 1997, Means and Smith, 1998). The things that identify community can also be those that marginalise people, such as being a poor, elderly, working-class person in an area full of wealthy middle-class people. Indeed, communities identify themselves as much by exclusion as inclusion, as we have seen in the reactions to refugees and asylum seekers in some towns in the UK. There is a risk of assuming that there is one simple meaning to *community*, under which all meanings can be collapsed. Hence it becomes easy to talk about 'the community' as if we knew what that meant, and 'community care' as a natural sequel to this understanding. The more we explore the meaning of *community*, the more we see that it does not necessarily possess the warm, fuzzy connotations it may at first have seemed to have. Much as in the way that, when we unpick notions of *family*, we find abuse, unhappiness and pain threaded through the rosy picture of closeness and love.

There is a risk of harking back to a 'Golden Age' of community which it is assumed has been lost in recent years. This myth persists despite the tendency for each generation to perceive the past as being organic and whole compared to the present (Payne, 1995; Means and Smith, 1998). Oral history studies reflect past understandings of community as being just as patchy and differentiated, as they are now, rather than demonstrating universal cohesion and mutual support (Bornat, 1997).

This leads us to question why, if *community* is such a contested notion, it has become so popular across the political spectrum as a basis for a system of care? We suggest the following reasons for this:

- Community care policies appealed to notions of personal responsibility in New Right ideology (latterly adopted by the New Left) and notions of collectivity in (primarily Old) Left ideology;
- Moves towards de-institutionalisation; and
- Reduction in public expenditure.

Hence, politicians and policy-makers bought into and fed the 'Golden Age' myth of community, one example being Prime Minister John Major's description of a 'spinster' cycling safely to church. Such warm, supportive notions of community were central to the debates about community care (Payne, 1995) although the realities of *community* are likely to be closer to the confusion and lack of cohesion we find when we examine Mr Trebus's situation.

What, then, are the implications of such notions of community as an unquestioned 'good thing' for the formulation of community care policies? Such policies appear to be based on premises which are, at worst, false and, at best, contested. We are likely to see a clash between rhetoric and reality, and continuing debates about what community care might mean in reality.

A lot has already been written about the background to, key thinking in and key messages from policy about community care and we have signposted further reading in these areas at the end of this chapter. The boxed text below serves as a summary. Issues of key thinking and influences behind the legislation will be addressed in detail in Chapter 2.

A Brief History of the development of community care policies 1962–93

1962   Enoch Powell, Minister of Health, announced his Hospital Plan, which launched the closure programme for large psychiatric hospitals and hospitals for people with learning disabilities. This marked a policy shift towards providing the bulk of care in the community, rather than in hospitals.

1968   The Seebohm Report (Seebohm Report, 1968) mentioned the need for greater emphasis to be placed on community, rather than institutional, care.

1970s   Little change. Two White Papers in this decade talked about a shift to community care, but there was no real political impetus for this.

1982   The Barclay Report (Barclay, 1982) focused on the community and the role of community social work.

1986   The Audit Commission (Audit Commission, 1986) emphasised the need for financial constraints on spending on residential care. At this time there was a *perverse incentive* for people to enter residential care because, for many, their fees were paid by the Department of Social Security (DSS) in Supplementary Benefit and they received much more than if they had remained at home (Audit Commission, 1986 p 4). The private home market was booming and there were also worries about the demographic changes that were pointing to an increase in the ageing population.

1988   The Griffiths Report (Griffiths,1988) made many recommen-dations about community care and was the final impetus for the legislation. It recommended that Social Services Departments (SSDs) would be the lead agencies in carrying out care management.

1989   The White Paper, *Caring for People* (DOH, 1989) gave the government's commitment to community care, to enable people *affected by problems of ageing, mental illness, mental handicap or physical or sensory disability to live as independently as possible in their own homes*.

1990   The NHS and Community Care Act implemented in April 1993.

Key thinking and influences behind the legislation:

- Large institutions no longer seen as the best way of caring for people and money tied up in institutional care was preventing funding of community care services. Community care would be a cheaper option.
- Concerns about excessive spending on welfare benefits, which was seen to be a drain on the economy.
- State provision of services was seen to be cumbersome, inflexible and unresponsive to need, fitting people to services which already existed and giving them little or no choice.
- New Right thinking in the 1980s saw the use of market forces as being the best way to operate public services.
- Growth of an increased managerial culture with emphasis on efficiency, economy and effectiveness.
- Growth of movements of people who use services and their carers voicing their views about services.
- Changes in attitudes towards empowering people who used services.
- Models of care management in use in the USA.

Key policy changes in community care in 1993

- Funds transferred from DSS (open-ended budget) to SSDs (capped budgets).
- Social Services and Health Authorities to produce community care plans.
- Social Services to be responsible for assessment and care management.
- Assessments to be needs-led, rather than service-driven, offering people a greater choice of services to meet their needs, and to enable them to stay in their own homes wherever feasible and sensible.
- Social Services to move from being a provider of services to an 'enabler' of service provision by:

  i)   Establishing a 'purchaser/provider' split;
  ii) Stimulating the development and provision of services by the private and not-for-profit sectors. Exemplified by the earmarking of 85 per cent of the transferred funds to be spent in these sectors;
  iii) Regulating providers through contracts;
  iv) Establishing 'arm's length' registration and inspection units;
  v)   Establishing complaints procedures;
  vi) New funding structure to achieve better value for money; and
  vii) Specific grants for mental illness.

Çore tasks in care management (SSI and SWSG, 1991a)

- Publishing information.
- Determining the level of assessment (screening).
- Assessing need.
- Care planning.
- Implementing the care plan.
- Monitoring.
- Reviewing.

Community care as care management

We have chosen to write extensively about care management, and particularly its impact on older people, in a book about community care. This is because we consider that the rhetoric of community care has been distorted to become the reality of care management. Care management has become the administrative and operational envelope for the operationalisation of community care policies (see Chapter 4). There are creative and imaginative approaches to working with people within their communities, and these have been developed both in theory (Smale *et al.*, 2000) and from consistent practical experience (Holman,1998; 2000). However, what we have witnessed in the UK since the implementation of the NHS and Community Care Act 1990 has been the development of an individualised care management model within mainstream Local Authority Social Services provision. Care management, as outlined in the box above and as described by Payne, has become *central to the implementation of community care policy in the 1990s* (Payne, 1997, p 277).

Care managers are the qualified and unqualified staff in social work and allied professions such as occupational therapy who are carrying out the task of care management. They are operating with dwindling resources and within the context of the political influences we noted above, and the societal changes we shall outline in Chapters 2 and 5. Following the transfer of funds for care in the community from the Department of Social Security to Local Authorities, care management for older people takes place generally, but not exclusively, within Local Authority settings.

As we shall discuss throughout the following chapters, the operation of community care as care management has had a profound impact on professionals working in the fields of health and social care, and on the organisational management of the settings in which they work. Above all, there has been a considerable impact on provision for people who use services and those who care for them.

Why this book, and who are these authors?

Writing this introduction, in a study knee-deep in books and papers about community care and care management, it's easy to ask the questions, 'Do we need another one?' and, 'What's different about this one?' To take the second question first: much, if not most, of what has been written about community care and care management has been written largely from a theoretical standpoint, drawing on theory about the nature of social work and the influence of social policy. We commend that, and, indeed, have used these texts in our research and throughout this book. By comparison, significantly less has been written from the basis of empirical research about the work of care managers although, again, we acknowledge the valuable work that has been done, and we have used this in our work.

Our claim to a standpoint which we see as rare in academic texts leads us to explain our biographies. Both authors are women who have worked with older people and so have seen the potential and actual impact of community care policies at first hand. Our respective interests in researching community care were prompted by our concerns for their effect on people such as those with whom we worked. Helen Gorman worked as a GP liaison social worker and Approved Social Worker (ASW) (Mental Health Act 1983), working with older people and people with mental ill-health, prior to taking up an academic post as a social work educator. Karen Postle was a social worker and later care manager in a team working with older people, and, more recently, worked with young disabled people. She is now a social work educator. Hence what we bring to this book is a combination of relevant and recent practice experience, knowledge gained from educating others, and the rigour of empirical research, conducted for doctoral study.

At a time when a lot was being written theoretically about community care and little from empirical studies, we both wanted to look much more closely at what was actually happening in care management. Our Ph.D. studies (Gorman, 1999b; and Postle, 1999) differ in their focus and methodologies. Both investigate the role of the care manager from the practitioner's perspective. They were carried out in different geographical locations within England: Gorman's in the Midlands, and Postle's in the South.

Gorman's work had two points of focus. It was an exploration into and an evaluation of the role of the care manager in the context of changing occupational identities and shifting professional boundaries. Further, it conducted a critical evaluation of the skills and knowledge required to perform that role in relation to the continuing professional education and development needs of those involved in complex care management. Her study, undertaken between 1995 and 1997, was based on a social constructivist approach that took the form of a survey of care managers from three Local Authorities, and thirty two long interviews conducted with individuals from that sample. The care managers, who were all designated as such by their employers, were based in Social Services Departments, hospital trusts, multidisciplinary teams within health trusts, community trusts, and one per cent from the voluntary sector. Gorman also completed a survey of post-qualifying students who had experience of care management, and conducted two focus group interviews with some of these alumni. The research approach was multi-method and involved data source triangulation (Denzin, 1994) and a robust form of data analysis using the QSR Nud*ist Qualitative Data Analysis Programme. Her thesis concluded that the prevailing orthodoxy of competency at the heart of professional identity was open to challenge, and that complex care management requires a corresponding contextual synthesis of knowledge and skill if it is to be of benefit to the people with whom care managers work.

Postle's thesis investigated whether the work of care managers working in Local Authority Social Services Departments has taken on attributes of a 'postmodern' contemporary society, and hence to what extent their work can be described by discourses of postmodernity. Her research was undertaken in two contrasting teams of care managers in Social Services area centres during 1996–7. Postle, like Gorman, used a constructivist approach, and her methodology comprised observations of and interviews with twenty care managers formerly designated as qualified or unqualified social workers working with older people, and their line managers. It included observation of 'in-house' training and a group discussion with 5 team managers. Interview and observation data was analysed using a grounded theory approach ensuring rigour (Glaser and Strauss, 1967; Lincoln and Guba, 1985; Guba and Lincoln, 1989). Postle concluded that that social work/care management is located in a transitional position between modernity and postmodernity, and displays characteristics of both states. The present implications of this position of professional uncertainty, both for care managers and for the older people with whom they work, led her to propose the need for a deconstruction and reconstruction of social work to meet the needs of older people. This has implications for research, training and practice.

So, in order to answer our first question about the need for another book about care management: we would argue that the authors' biographies and the nature of our research enable us to make a unique contribution to the debate about the transitional nature of community care as operationalised in care management.

What the book aims to do

Our aims are as follows:

- To draw on literature and our respective research studies to give an accurate reflection of the current picture of care management work, reflecting on the impact of this practice for staff and, crucially and inextricably linked to this, for service users.

- Debates abound concerning what is meant by the nature of 'evidence-based practice' highlight that there is a risk that this can become interpreted solely as the province of positivist, quantitative methodologies. We therefore present our work, based on rigorously conducted qualitative research, as pertinent and timely evidence in debates about care management/community care.

- Acknowledging that community care is in transition, we seek to determine what the potential for its development, encompassing threats and opportunities, might be.

Outline of the book

Chapter 2 outlines the origins of and influences on care management. It explores the evolution of community care as care management and the impact of managerialism within the context of diminished resources. In discussing the changing role of social workers, the chapter addresses their de-professionalisation and the commodification of their labour. Notions of partnership, often taken as a given in the community care reforms, are examined critically. The chapter ends by questioning the likely future of community care, with both optimistic and pessimistic insights.

In Chapter 3 we examine whether care management does indeed provide any care or any management. The nature of care management work is discussed, highlighting the change in the nature of the work to one that entails increased bureaucracy and decreased use of self. We question the impact of this on the people with whom care managers work and, indeed, the likely future role of social work if such changes continue. In discussing how care managers 'manage' people's care, we question the short-termist, individualised nature of care management and outline prerequisites for change.

Chapter 4 moves to look at the nature of decision-making in community care and explores the influences on decision-making about who gets a service. The societal context of care managers' decision-making is discussed, and approaches to inter-disciplinary working are examined to ascertain whether these are likely to lead to better decisions for service users. Examples of decision-making dilemmas are given to highlight the complexity of issues facing care managers in their work. Issues of accountability are outlined and their relevance to care managers' autonomy discussed. The lack of any link between community care/care management and strategies for community development are shown as being all too apparent. The chapter concludes that there is greater need for reflection in care management, and for transparency in the decision-making processes.

In Chapter 5 we explore the complex nature of empowerment before exploring, with the help of examples from research, whether care management offered opportunities for empowerment strategies. We conclude that these opportunities are limited, and that care managers are finding increasingly that their work is de-skilling and demoralising. As in Chapter 2, we consider the implications of a demoralised workforce on the service users with whom they work, concluding that disempowered workers are unlikely to empower others. We end with consideration of some possible strategies for empowerment.

We reach our conclusions in Chapter 6, identifying threats in the continuation of care management work which include reductionist practices commodifying the emotional labour of care managers' work and a real risk of the 'NVQisation' of professional skill to the detriment of service users. We emphasise the need for the continuing personal and professional development of staff engaged in promoting the independence of older people through care management. There are rays of hope where there is scope for preventative work and creative, collaborative partnerships with service users. A shift in the nature of work within communities may, sadly, come too late for Mr Trebus, but we hope that any such shift will have regard for the art of professional social work in its many forms.

Throughout the book quotations from care management staff and summaries of work observed are taken from primary data quoted in our respective doctoral research (Gorman 1999b, and Postle 1999) unless stated otherwise .

Postscript
Sadly, as this book was going to press, we learnt that Mr Trebus had died. The final months of his life were spent in a residential care home. People who had known him remembered his eccentricity, wit and tenacity.

Edmund Zygfryd Trebus 11th November 1918 – September 29th 2002

Suggested background reading:
Bornat, J, Johnson, J, Pereira, C, Pilgrim, D and Williams, F (eds) (1997) *Community Care: a Reader* London, Macmillan
Cowen, H (1999) *Community Care, Ideology and Social Policy* Hemel Hempstead, Prentice Hall Europe
Means, R and Smith, R (1998) *Community Care Policy and Practice* (2nd edn) London, Macmillan
Payne, M (1995) *Social Work and Community Care* London, Macmillan
Sharkey, P (2000) *The Essentials of Community Care: a guide for practitioners* London, Macmillan
Wilson, G (ed) (1995) *Community Care: Asking the Users* London, Chapman & Hall

Chapter 2
Origins and Influences

The development of care management

The term 'community care' is used generically to cover a multiplicity of realities. For those at the receiving end of care services, much of the current reality is about eligibility for services and whether needs will be met. For those involved in implementing community care on a professional basis the reality of community care is the completion of documentation with an eye on monitoring mechanisms in the context of limited resources. How do the concepts inherent in the notion of community care discussed in Chapter 1 fit with these scenarios? In 1965 Titmus described community care as 'an everlasting cottage garden trailer'. Rather like a vine, it has had good seasons and bad ones – for the pessimist, it may appear that the vine that held so much promise may never come to fruition but for the optimist the best may be yet to come!

This chapter will evaluate critically some of the influences on the development of community care in the UK since the 1970s. A revolution took place during this period that transmuted the notion of community care into the systems of care management dominating the way that care is offered and delivered. There are a number of influences that have had a fundamental effect on the way that care is experienced by the majority of service users at the beginning of the twenty-first century. Care management as the main expression of community care existed in a nascent form even before the Seebohm reforms of the early 1970s. The social workers who belonged to the new generic social service departments at that time would not have used the term 'care management', but they did engage in a process of assessment, care planning, implementation and evaluation. However, the way that social workers carried out their work was to change in the wake of the Conservative Government's vision of community care expressed in *Caring for People* (DOH, 1989). The NHS and Community Care Act 1990 and the subsequent Department of Health/Social Services Inspectorate documentation set the tone of reforms of the early 1990s that continue to dominate the way that care in the community is constructed in the UK. The 1990 Act was not only concerned with differing philosophies about the best way to provide care, it was also concerned fundamentally with the organising and financing of services. The focus of the reforms was a mixed economy of care that would increase choice for consumers through introducing market principles into welfare. At the same time the reduction of the power of the welfare bureaucracy (no bad thing in the eyes of many users of services) was to take the form of a shift from monopolistic providers to enablers and purchasers of care services. This, in turn, would have an impact on the role of those whose functions were circumscribed by agency: the managers, social workers, nurses, and home care and residential staff. What happened during this period changed the way that social service organisations were managed, the way that social workers and health professionals did their work, and, most importantly, how those who received services and their informal carers experienced the translation of community care into care-managed activity.

Several key themes emerged during the last two decades of the twentieth-century that built on policy trends of earlier decades; one such theme was the move away from institutional care to care at home provided by informal carers and public and voluntary services. The transfer of responsibility for health and social care to localities continues with the development of Primary Care Groups and their evolution into Care Trusts. The policy thrust of devolution is driven in part by a finite budget for public health. Hence it could be argued that community care and primary care, as a manifestation of that devolution, become one potential solution to an insoluble dilemma related to maintaining a 'welfare state' in the UK.

Some of the dichotomies in providing public care services continued to be significant in the way that care in the community took shape following the community care reforms of the 1990s and have a bearing on how it continues to be viewed. There are five interrelated key themes that will be identified in this chapter and are echoed throughout the book. These are:

- Care management as a distortion of community care;
- From new managerialism to best value;
- From social worker to care manager – the demise of the professional?;
- The search for quality and the realities of audit; and
- The 'mantra' of partnership – is it workable?

Is care management a distortion of community care?
In the USA in the 1980s, with no history of state provision, case management was envisaged by some as gate-keeping with an emphasis on cost containment, an answer to fragmented services and partial funding from insurance companies. Although it only proved to be cost-effective under certain limited conditions (Dant and Gearing, 1990), it was this notion of cost containment and the concept of the management of services that fired the imagination of the policy-makers in the UK and was to make an impact on a UK welfare system in the 1990s. Despite the differences between the US 'non-system' and the complex welfare system existing in the UK, parallel approaches were encouraged. The appeal of a care management system to the Conservative

Government of the day lay in an approach that emphasised outcomes and concentrated on the financial aspects of care and the need for effective targeting of resources. The Griffiths Report (Griffiths, 1988), however, emphasised that the potential strength of a care management system was the value of co-ordination and the delivery of a seamless services to users in the community, preferably in their own homes.

The term 'care management' emerged as common parlance in health and welfare settings in the late 1980s following *Caring for People* (DOH, 1989). Huxley (1993) refers to the semantic and linguistic engineering of the term *case* management into *care* management in the UK Department of Health reforms of this period. The distinction between these two terms remains a critical issue for care management in this country. This dichotomy may be seen as the difference between the managerial and administrative control of care services and the meeting of the individual care needs of those who require care in the community, perhaps through 'casework' intervention. Care management (as it was to be defined by the government through *Caring for People* (DOH, 1989), the NHS and Community Care Act 1990, and subsequent practice and policy guidance) was conceptualised as an administrative model within a consumerist framework. This approach fitted in with the growing emphasis on the 'market' in welfare and the idea that people could choose from a range of services that included those provided by the private and voluntary sectors.

The community care policy embedded in the NHS and Community Care Act 1990, and the policy and practice guidance that followed, obliged Social Services Departments to make changes to three areas of their functions:

- to establish new care management systems that would be needs-led, including new procedures for assessment;
- to become enablers rather than providers of services, which meant involvement with independent providers and the separation of purchaser and provider functions within social services departments; and
- to establish more effective joint planning with other agencies through strategic community care plans.

The government of the day had a clear agenda related to cost containment and the reduction of public provision of services and privatisation, yet in the early 1990s there was no clear idea about what care management meant and who should be care-managed. Early pilot projects (Challis and Davies, 1986) were useful, but advocated a form of care management that was finely tuned and did not necessarily fit with a wider process of change that was affecting local authorities at the time. Local authorities, faced with demands to get an assessment system in place by April 1993 and to publish strategic care plans for their areas in conjunction with other relevant organisations, concentrated on developing these aspects rather than giving sufficient thought to the whole process of care management (Lewis and Glennester, 1996) and an integrated strategy for care in the community. Different models of operation were possible (Hudson, 1993; Øvretveit, 1993), connected to the way that local authorities embraced the purchaser/provider split. The government argued that if the service was to respond to need, assessment should be separated from service provision (SSI and SWSG, 1991c). Early evaluation research on the implementation of care management picked up an emphasis on a job rather than a process, with a corresponding impact on existing roles as well as newly-defined roles (DOH and Challis, 1994).

The UK White Paper *Caring for People* (DOH, 1989) described assessment and case management as the cornerstones of community care, and the Audit Commission referred to it as the 'lynch pin'. Care management became then, and has remained, the point at which welfare objectives and resource constraints are closest together. Much depends upon the coherence, form, style and structure of the care management processes implemented and the level of budgetary control imposed. Variations in care management systems to date have depended on a number of features (DOH and Challis, 1994: DOH/SSI, 1998) and patterns of resource allocation within authorities:

- local organisational structures;
- the local context of implementation and local government reorganisations;
- local expectation of service systems in terms of the degree of separation between purchaser and provider;
- the extensiveness of a local mixed economy;
- the presence of substitute and complementary services
- the perceived goals of care management in terms of seamless services for users; and
- relationships with health providers.

From new managerialism to best value
'New managerialism' was more than just shaking up social services to make them more responsive to better management. It involved a fundamental change in the way the work carried out by social workers was configured: it shifted the agenda from a notion of professional work to one where the dominating agenda was management structures and practices. This theme will be expressed in a variety of ways throughout this book.

Those working in the public services since the early 1980s have experienced a continuous period of change. Some writers have argued that social work takes place in a context of postmodernity (Parton, 1996a), and while this is described as a contentious issue there is nonetheless some indication that the nature of 'change' itself has changed. It is now experienced frequently as random and directionless (Bauman, 1992). This process has been captured in various discourses, ranging from the macro to the micro, such as globalisation, post-Fordism, the post-bureaucratic organisation, the new public management, and the mixed economy of welfare, plus a variety of terms that relate to the role of the state itself, such as the contract state, the enabling state and the managerial state (Clarke and Newman, 1997). Most of the postwar generation of citizens grew up with the notion that the welfare state was a 'safety net', a reassurance that people would be cared for in old age or in bad times, despite the reality that care was dispensed through a bureaucracy that had since the Poor Law days distinguished between the 'deserving' and the 'undeserving'. The realities of the welfare state have been tied up with the welfare bureaucracy and the notion of public service. Stewart and Walsh (1992) identify several assumptions underlying the culture of public service:

- An assumption of self-sufficiency – that a public organisation responsible for a function will carry out the function directly;
- Direct control is exercised via supervision through a hierarchy;
- An assumption of uniformity – a service provided should be on a uniform basis within the jurisdiction of the organisation;
- Accountability of public servants to those who receive a service is through the political process; and
- Standardised recruitment and staffing policies.

The emphasis was on the traditions of administration, hierarchy and professionalism, bound up with collectivised notions of equity, justice and impartiality. This notion of the welfare bureaucracy was to change with the development of the 'new managerialism'.

The term 'quasi-market' that formed part of the new managerialist agenda meant the separation of state finance from state provision and the introduction of competition for provision from independent agencies (Le Grand and Bartlett, 1993). The state could be conceived as 'contracting' in the sense that it was no longer a sole provider, while at the same time 'contracting' with the voluntary and private sector in agreements to provide services for those deemed to be in need of services; it had become a 'contracting state' (Harden, 1992). The reform of community care highlighted the perceived need for a split between purchasing and providing responsibilities, the development of forms of contract between purchasers and providers, a concern for services to be based on need rather than resources available, the delegation of authority for budget control, and the pursuit of choice through provider competition. Clarke and Newman (1997) identify the impact of the new managerialism in terms of attempts to realign a series of relationships, between the state and the citizen, between the state and the economy, and between the state and its organisational forms, including labour processes. New managerialism encapsulates the belief that social problems embodied in the need for community care can be solved by the better management of resources, including human resources. This continues to be a valid discourse in a critical evaluation of the Labour Government's 'third way' (Giddens, 1994), and in terms of the development of the concept of 'best value'. In theory, the delivery by local authorities of the local services that people want, to the quality they want and at the price they are prepared to pay is the hallmark of the 'best value' strategy. The market and the notion of competition remains a central part of the strategy linked to the belief that, through competition and comparing performance, better quality services will emerge.

The development of the market in health and social care in the form of the purchaser/provider split meant that, in the 1990s, Social Services Departments became enablers rather than providers of services, with staff in some local authorities being required to elect to work in either the provider side or the purchaser side of the organisation. The idea of 'consumer sovereignty' – that is, that users have free choices about the services they can have – is limited within care management because the nature of the relationship with the state is one in which there are controls set by the Social Services Department through eligibility criteria and restrictions in resources (Wistow *et al.*, 1994). Furthermore, these controls are fundamental to the way in which the care manager who usually defines 'the need' has to operate. Consumers may express their opinions and exercise their bounded rights, yet the discourse with the consumer is predefined by the organisation through its management. Inevitably choice is restricted if users need services that they cannot purchase on the open market as independent purchasers. In some respects consumerist notions such as flexibility and innovation have some relevance, yet the lack of redress for poor-quality service, the lack of overt critical standards and the constraints of working with limited budgets appear to belie notions of consumerism, which then appear to be superficial.

Market changes came hand-in-hand with increased 'managerialism' within health and social care agencies that had value for money auditing as one of their main characteristics. Power (1997) describes four possible operationalisations of the concept of accountability – fiscal regularity, economy (value for money), efficiency and effectiveness. He comments that through this 'new managerialism', the audit explosion had become accepted as part of the quality control processes in health settings. In order to effect such changes, standards had to be defined and practice observed, and such observations compared with defined standards so that activity could be evaluated with the aim of improvement. Within Social Services Departments the control of quality through audit tended to be confined initially to certain areas of activity such as the registration and inspection of residential care. However, with the growth of care management stimulated by the purchaser/provider split and the development of an administrative/managerial culture, the scene was set for a further intensification of the 'quality' process and the need for evaluation of practice as part of that overall strategy. The notion of audit and the significance of the monitoring of performance at work through the achievement of targets became part of the Labour Government's strategy for the reform of Health and Social Services through its 'modernising' agenda (DOH, 1998a; DOH, 1998c; DOH, 2000a; DOH, 2000b).

The demonstration of a commitment to the quality process depends on creating attitudes of creativity and independence in the workforce (Townsend and Gebhardt, 1990), characteristics that had become subsumed within a new managerialist agenda that embraced a market approach to welfare and contested previously-held notions of professionalism. New managerialism had an impact on relationships between both the manager and the professional worker, and the consumer and the professional worker, in the context of the welfare project. The notion of health and social care as commodities that could be purchased and could be chosen from a range of alternatives can be critiqued as a chimera concealing a reality that incorporates risk management and the balance between autonomy and control. Various dichotomies exist relating to the balance between care and control in the exercise of care management, one of those being the balance of power between the welfare professional and the user of the service, and the other being autonomy of the welfare professional in his or her role within the bureaucracy. These ideas will be developed more fully in Chapter 4.

A lack of confidence in public sector care, the development of welfare pluralism, a market in health and social care and the growth of managerialism have provided fertile ground for the growth of anti-professionalism in general and anti-social work in particular, sentiments that did not diminish with the arrival of a Labour government. Conflicts arise when decisions have to be taken about the quality of life of others that reflect the interpretation of social care as a commodity with users of services configured as 'consumers' of welfare. From the perspective of care managers, who are usually professionally qualified as social workers, there would be an expectation that they have some professional autonomy in their role and that they may act as advocates for the user, thus acting in the users' best interests in securing the best care available (Brandon and Hawkes, 1998). Yet the reality has been that the many changes experienced by those working in the welfare system of the UK has minimised the consideration of values issues in favour of getting the job done to meet targets set by a management agenda. Fundamental values such as mutuality (interpreted by Holman (1993) as the recognition of mutual obligations for others stemming from a common notion of kinship in which material reward is not the major force), appears to have skewed the idea of 'community care' to mean an individual care compact that is influenced openly and strongly by managerial controls. This has affected the work of social workers in community care, and for some commentators has led to a lack of recognition of the richness of human diversity, a point raised as a significant issue by Hadley and Clough (1996) in their case studies of social care workers' views of work prior to and during the community care reforms.

From professional social worker to the occupation of care manager?
An important feature of any discussion about the role of the care manager is the notion of the state mediated professional (Johnson, 1972), an analysis that emphasises that authority exists through power bestowed by the state. Many of the dilemmas experienced by care managers (Gorman, 1999b; Postle, 1999) relate to tensions between autonomy and accountability in the exercise of their role. To follow Johnson's argument of power relations and therefore control (bound up with who mediates in the producer/consumer relationship, and who defines needs and how they should be met), it would appear that the care manager is potentially in a position of power. Yet the current context of welfare is one of fewer resources and devolution of responsibility with centralised control over resources. In general, consumers as users of social care are unlikely to participate in the co-production of welfare as citizens. Rather, they are being forced to choose between the services on offer despite a policy rhetoric about the meeting of needs (Wilson, 1995).

Running parallel with the growth of government guidelines and procedures, and a formalising of activities and roles within a bureaucracy, there has been a circumscription of professional autonomy and discretion. The introduction of a market approach to care with a parallel rise in consumerism, with the social work 'client' (albeit a problematic term) being referred to as 'consumer', 'customer' or 'user', denotes a shift to a market-based relationship with rights to certain services and rights to complain being stated. This implies, or at least does not question, an assumption that clients of Social

Services are customers or consumers in the same way as those of, for example, a shop or hotel, and does not consider the complex and contested notion of commodification of welfare (Baldock and Ungerson, 1994; Phillips, 1996; Fawcett and Featherstone, 1998). In the context of care management the relationships with clients are placed on a different footing: consumers can use complaints procedures and seek a Judicial Review because the relationship is bound by market forces and by an increased emphasis on conflicting imperatives, choice and adversarial approaches. This is a challenge to a 'professional' relationship based on expertise and trust, and in a sense reinforces mediative control. These forces appear to have had their greatest effect in community care, and more specifically in adult services, particularly in the care of disabled people (Mandelstam and Schwehr, 1995). The well-known Barry judgment (*R* v. *Gloucestershire County Council ex parte Barry* (1997)) emphasised not only that social services could take resources into account when meeting service users' needs, but also reinforced the significance of the interpretation of eligibility criteria in every case that involves assessment for community care services. Challenges to social services decisions made by care managers regularly hit the headlines in the press, and make it imperative that staff are mindful of the complexity of policy and practice guidelines that relate to decision-making about community care services.

The role of the care manager as state functionary is a dominant paradigm and bears a direct relationship to the transformation of the social work role into that of the care manager in work with adults in the community. The crisis of social work, which has existed for decades, has once again been highlighted by shifts within the organisational framework that supports it as an activity. Satyamurti (1981), writing in the context of post-Seebohm Report reorganisations in the social services, saw the crisis as emanating less from changes in the work itself than from the social workers' relationships with that work and their interpretations of what they were doing. The new situation, stimulated by the community care reforms, threw into relief and made more glaringly obvious situations that had hitherto been present, such as obstacles to providing an effective service for clients and the intensification of control functions, even though they may have been reconfigured in a different way from before. In the context of contemporary care management, however, a claim could be made that the work itself has changed in terms of the functions of the care manager, related directly to changed paradigms of welfare economics. Such a fundamental shift impinges upon how welfare work is conceived, organised and managed. There are a number of contradictions in care management that reflect the changing nature of welfare work. These include:

- the relationship between care management as an administrative strategy and care management as therapeutic intervention;
- a diversity of models for implementation;
- the relationship between the process of care management and its outcomes;
- the concept of individualism in the context of systems complexity;
- risk management in a climate of limited resources and raised expectations; and
- the relationship between care management and activity considered by many to be professional work.

These themes, which will be developed more fully throughout this book, can be viewed as tensions implicit in the many, and occasionally divergent, policy directives issued by the Department of Health and the Social Services Inspectorate over a number of years, and that in turn have shaped professional services for community care (Kelly, 1998).

Johnson's (1972) 'state-mediated' professional is central to the discussion, particularly Johnson's theory that occupational control and power relations are bound up with who mediates in the producer/consumer relationship, and who defines needs and the way they should be met. Social work is located mainly within the hierarchical, bureaucratic structures of local government (Howe, 1986, Clough; 1990, Hugman, 1991a), yet social workers themselves have at times been reluctant to accept the notion of professionalism, or have positively rejected it (Bailey and Brake, 1975). The care manager has to make decisions in risky and problematic situations, thus emphasising the use of appropriate judgement in the context of the assessment, planning, co-ordination and implementation of a package of care. The expertise of the state-mediated professional has been redefined in the context of the marketisation of social services, and shifted social work with adults away from an historical emphasis on service and altruism.

Care managers are mainly qualified social workers, although they can be workers from related professional groups such as nurses or occupational therapists working in a social services context, and in some authorities non-qualified staff act as care managers. In most social work interventions the state mediates the tasks of the social worker, both in terms of who is recognised as a client, and what resources are available to help ameliorate the problems recognised by eligibility for a service. Compliance in the role of social worker is influenced strongly by supervision, with some perceived professional autonomy in the role, and as much loyalty to that professional identity as allegiance to status as a local authority employee. Social work, perceived as ' doing good', is part of a philanthropic and liberating ethos which has been a significant influence on social work practice for a number of decades and has formed part of the skills of social work taught on social work training courses. These factors remain significant in the way that social workers who are now care managers view their current employment. However, as Hugman (1991a) reminds us, altruism has been bound up with the notion of the 'subordinate' client as part of a complex web of power dynamics. The social worker would perceive of him/herself as 'doing what is to the best of his/her knowledge correct,' (Davies, 1983) based on the skills and values of social work, but with an awareness of the need to follow the rules as set down through policy and practice guidance derived from the state and interpreted by the Local Authority. For most social workers there would be an expectation of an element of autonomy in handling cases, as engagement with clients is largely on an individual basis. Payne (1996) explores definitions of social work, acknowledging a range of dichotomies related to social work as a profession within social work agencies, one such dilemma being the promotion of reflexive and therapeutic perspectives that emphasise autonomous professional activity with a strong ethical base within agencies that limit autonomy because of the impact of political, bureaucratic and social control. In general terms, differences in approach can be categorised, from Payne 1998, as:

- individualist/reformist, workers taking their functions from defined responsibilities and the role of their agencies;

- reflexive/therapeutic that has a focus on helping individuals to achieve personal growth; and

- socialist/collective approaches that emphasise changed structures in society to combat unfairness and the creation of alliances through shared problems.

The Local Authority social work role in community care has been focused largely on the first category listed, with some reference to therapeutic intervention, although this has diminished considerably over the years. There has been a distinct lack of community development activity on the part of paid professionals despite the rhetoric of encouraging user participation in community care planning. However, the development of the notion of the 'broker' of services, particularly in care management with people who have physical disabilities, is a significant shift in perspective, representing a clear challenge to concepts of dependency and reinforcing the politics of participation in the social disability movement (Oliver, 1990). These developments are a challenge to public bureaucracy and the state mediation of care in the community, and to professional roles within health and welfare agencies.

The Direct Payments Act 1996 offers a bounded opportunity for some users to organise and pay for their own care as exemplified by Brandon and Hawkes (1998) and Clark and Spafford (2001). These rights have now been extended to older people (DOH, 1998b) and may prove to be a positive way forward to enhancing independence for a greater number of service users if a creative and empowering approach is taken towards service users' rights (see Chapter 5). Similarly, creative use of the Prevention Grant (DOH, 1998b) has potential for use in the development of community services.

The drive to achieve quality becomes problematic in a context where there are tensions between the individualised care of someone in need and the complexity of welfare systems operating in a climate of limited resources. Decisions have to be made about eligibility for services that relate to interpretations of law and policy around eligibility and rationing, local demands and priorities, and the orientation of the care manager in terms of personal and professional identity. In the assessment of risk as well as the assessment for services leading to a package of care for an individual, painful decisions have to be made and people will not get what they want, either because of lack of resources or because their needs conflict with those of others (Smale *et al.*, 1993).

The search for quality and the realities of audit

There are several policy themes outlined in various contemporary government documents (DOH, 1998b; DOH, 2000a; DOH, 2000b) that have an impact on a discussion of quality in community care. These can be summarised as:

- a policy drive to review services;
- the promotion of relationships (both between service users and service providers and between agencies and workers charged with the task of providing planned care in the community); and
- the need to develop a skilled workforce.

There is a range of inherent contradictions and tensions in these themes that are interlinked. Government policy has become bounded increasingly by the audit and monitoring of work activity. The underlying aim of finding ways to improve outcomes for service users is laudable, and would be shared by the vast majority both as citizens and workers in the public sector, but the means being used to justify the ends require some critique.

While it may be acceptable at certain levels of work for a judgement of competence to be the 'gold standard' to allow workers to practice in certain contexts and settings, an assumption that the existence of basic standards of technology necessarily means that quality work has been delivered is erroneous. This is particularly so in work that requires interpersonal interaction and the demonstration of care and respect for individuals (Dissenbacher, 1989). A baseline that emphasises technical skills and denies the realities of emotional labour, rather than setting a gold standard, can be influential in encouraging poor-quality work (Gorman, 2000b). The job can be done to standards, but the carrying out of the work may not necessarily improve outcomes as perceived by the recipients of those services.

Much of the previous discussion is linked to interpretations of the notion of quality and this is a theme that is developed throughout this book. The concept of total quality management aims to improve the effectiveness of organisations through involving everyone in a process of improvement (Oakland, 1989). The emphasis in this approach is on holism and the importance of recognising both process and outcome. However, as Gaster (1995) points out, in the context of public welfare there will generally be a gap between what is desirable if all aspects of quality were to be measured, and the reality of what can actually be achieved with existing resources and levels of commitment. There is nothing wrong with trying to measure quality; the problem comes in the acceptance that any measure is unlikely to be perfect and is subject to a number of constraints. The use of performance measures as tools of censure rather than as aids to development compounds the problem. The relevance of the quality agenda to training needs and the 'competence' of staff will be discussed fully in the final chapter.

The mantra of partnership – is it working?
If we say it often enough, may we believe it is happening? Partnership has become the 'in' word and everyone is meant to be doing it. The notion of partnership with users and inter-agency work to provide seamless services has been a consistent theme throughout the reforms of the 1990s and has re-emerged in the modernising agenda of the Labour Government. Despite the attempts to put inter-agency work and collaborative working practices between health and social services staff high on the agenda, it is possible to trace a number of 'realities' that have emerged from the rhetoric. From the outset, the plans and possibilities set out in the Griffiths Report (1988) incorporated policy contradictions related to the creation of a market in welfare that would in turn affect work roles and relationships between the face-workers, service-users and the agencies. Competition and collaboration are uneasy bedfellows. To get people to work together for the better good of others in a climate of competition requires an attitudinal shift as well as the existence of favourable systems that allow such developments to flourish. Repeating the mantra of working together without understanding the real meaning of partnership, or presuming that you can locate a group of people

in the same place and assume they will work together is a naïve assumption, but one that has been common in misunderstanding the complexities of inter-professional work. In many ways the existence of the notion since the early 1990s in government documents may lead us to assume that genuine partnership work is the norm. This contrasts with understandings of collaborative working that offer hope for better outcomes for people using services (Beresford and Trevillion, 1995; Payne, 2000)

A lack of understanding about the purpose and direction of inter-professional and inter-agency work and limitations on a consistent training commitment has hampered many developments that held promise. At the same time there have been examples of collaborative projects that *have* worked: for example, the Birmingham Community Care Special Action Project (Barnes and Wistow, 1995) and CAIPE (UK Centre for the Advancement of Interprofessional Education), an organisation that has offered a consistent critique of collaborative endeavour whilst encouraging positive and innovative change towards 'working together' (Barr, 1994). Yet the use of the term 'partnership' in the context of welfare in general, and care management in particular, is problematic. The term 'collaboration' and a notion of 'going over to the enemy' implies the possibility of conflict and the resolution of this to reach a state of collaboration (Gorman, 2000a). The term 'partnership' with its implications of sharing, joint contribution and a degree of intimacy seems out of place in a context of the realities of care management as expressed in this chapter, where eligibility criteria, audit and administrative control dominate to the exclusion of personal interaction and community involvement. Such dilemmas will be expanded upon in Chapters 4 and 5.

Conclusion

Attempts have been made by the Labour Government in power to free up some of the systems blockages to joint funding that marred collaborative effort in service provision (Health Act 1999). Problems that have haunted successful partnership work still exist, however, with the drive for competition to raise standards (best value) running alongside partnership arrangements between agencies, and the recognition of the voice of the user running alongside the realities of power and control in resource allocation. A positive interpretation of 'best value' means flexibility and putting local people first. A tension still remains between strengthening local democracy by councils taking full account of the views of local people, and the drive to satisfy central government's criteria or those of external auditors. The implementation of the Human

Rights Act 1998 could ensure that practitioners and managers are mindful of good practice requirements relating to the voice of the user.

It may be that community care expressed as Titmus's 'cottage garden trailer' is on the brink of rejuvenation. The modernising agenda that includes *The New NHS* (DOH, 1997) and *Modernising Social Services* (DOH, 1998b), with its emphasis on partnership, local involvement and quality expressed as people's needs, are positive indicators of a renewal in the meaning of care in the community. Major problems remain, however. The legacy of the past may continue to haunt the future. A quiet revolution took place in the late 1980s and early 1990s that altered fundamentally the way that care in the community was envisioned. The market in health and social care is likely to remain, and a return to a system of comprehensive public health and welfare unlikely. Systems of care management became the embodiment of care in the community as experienced by millions of people in this country who needed help to maintain themselves in their own homes. The struggle to match resources to needs will continue, but, unlike the world of the 1970s, the conflicts are much more in the public eye and open to legal challenge.

Chapter 3
Any care or any management?

Introduction: a letter to the editor

I am 80 years old and live alone. I was briefly in hospital for an operation on my hand and was visited by social services who asked if there was any help I would need when I went home. Yes, I replied, someone to bathe me and clean the house. These things are not possible, she said. They are not insured for bathing clients and cleaning was limited to 'dusting the tops', no furniture could be moved. How awful it must be to be disabled and dependent on social services – never to have a bath, and never to have the dust cleaned out from behind your chair or under your bed. Do people realise what care in the community amounts to? (Letter to the Guardian from Barbara Hutton, August 2000)

Quoting this letter, we can imagine the response from the hard-pressed staff in Local Authority Social Services offices:

We have to stick to eligibility criteria and we can only meet category 1.

We don't do anything except personal care any more. We just don't have the resources.

Bathing is such a risk in case someone gets injured. Nurses used to do it but they don't any more.

People's expectations of what they can get have been raised and we just can't meet them.

While we acknowledge the problems staff are facing, we think that Barbara Hutton's question *Do people realise what care in the community amounts to?* is valid, timely and pertinent, and we would speculate that, like her, many people do not realise what community care does, or all too frequently does *not*, amount to until they or someone they know experiences difficulties. Having outlined the political, ideological and societal context for community care in Chapter 2, we noted that questions remain concerning the extent to which community care was care 'in' or 'by' the community. Over time it appears that there has been a reinforcement of state control of the organisation and allocation of care, and this has been magnified by the care management process. This chapter looks at the reality of community care in practice. It questions whether the operation of 'care management' contains much in the way of either care or management, and suggests that questioning current practice may be the first step on the road to finding approaches to community care which might better meet the needs of the people who use services.

Social worker to care manager – a changed role?

It had been envisaged that the introduction of care management would inevitably change the role of social work staff who undertook the task. Following implementation of the NHS and Community Care Act 1990 in April 1993, much research focused on the changed role of the social worker and the sense of loss of social work skills (for example, see Henwood, 1995; Rachman, 1995). The counselling/therapy role that care managers might have undertaken as part of their work was unclear. This resulted in a worrying trend as some social workers dealt with what they perceived as a loss or under-use of their therapeutic skills by leaving the profession to work as therapists (Hirst, 1995). This echoes the situation in America, where the growth of individualised therapeutic work, coupled with financial rewards for this and the difficulties of working in a reluctant welfare state, has caused social workers to leave their profession for the more lucrative work of therapy (Specht and Courteney, 1994). Care management was similarly seen as squeezing out the less quantifiable skills of social workers, such as emotional support and counselling, and replacing them with bureaucratic and mechanistic approaches involving heavy caseloads and increased administrative tasks (Hoyes *et al.*, 1994; Parton, 1996a).

So what do care managers now spend their time doing? This is how one care manager described what takes up most of his time:

> *Contracts, paperwork, writing assessments ... writing assessments is OK ... If you look at setting a care package up you've got to write an assessment, got to work out which agencies you're talking about, got to write out an initial service contract. If they're going into respite care, into a rest home, then you're talking about residential contracts. You can have two initial service contracts if you can't get one agency to do the whole lot.*

His comments typified what most care managers described about dealing with bureaucratic tasks largely related to contractual arrangements (Postle, 1999). Much, if not most, of care managers' time is now taken up with paperwork (Lewis and Glennester, 1996; Lewis *et al.*, 1997; Webb *et al.*, 1998).

Care managers attributed the increased bureaucracy to the operation of the market and increased budgetary constraints. The notion of an internal market resulting in a purchaser/provider split, however operated (Means and Smith, 1998), has introduced new ways of working for care managers. They had previously used their 'in house' services which required little paperwork and only a very simple means test to calculate the amount people paid for domiciliary or residential care. They commented that using the market to purchase domiciliary and residential care had brought benefits in terms of flexibility of care provision, but also disadvantages such as wide variety in quality of service provided, with some agencies' standards declining if, for example, they took on too much work. In terms of the changed nature of the care managers' work, operating in a market for care has involved them in a plethora of procedures and contractual arrangements with care agencies and residential homes, as shown in the care manager's comments.

Additionally, the care manager quoted above described the charging policy forms that had to be completed:

You've also got to do the charging policy stuff so you've got to do financial assessments for the charging policy. When the package is set up you've got to inform the financial department so that they can initiate the charging process ... So an assessment and writing up an assessment is over half a day ... a maximum two hours with the client, then at least half a day... [the bureaucracy's about] managing finances ... as the care manager, you're responsible for the first part of that, getting everything into those financial systems.

Most Local Authorities are working with very restricted resources, and have introduced charging policies to ensure that people contribute to the cost of their care. Care managers were responsible for obtaining details of finances from their clients in order to calculate what the person had to pay for their care (Postle, 1999). Although the finance section arranged for payments to be made, if anomalies or queries arose, cases were passed back to care managers for clarification or to obtain more information. While there is clearly a need for accountability regarding public funds, the result of undertaking extensive financial enquiries was that care managers became further embroiled in bureaucratic tasks. This was in addition to the administration of means testing which exacerbates poverty and social exclusion (Bradley and Manthorpe, 1997; McLeod and Bywaters, 2000).

The health of elderly people with whom care managers work is often precarious, necessitating frequent changes in their care needs. Care is bought on individual contracts for people and therefore changes – such as admission to hospital – necessitate alterations to care plans and contracts. The care manager quoted below found that she could keep up with initial contracts but was very concerned about coping with the innumerable 'temporary adjustments' which had to be completed whenever a person's care changed:

It's the admin side of it. I think I'm in favour of care management. I think it's good for the client, but it's not social work as such ... I don't like paperwork. I think I've come to not mind filling in contracts and arrangements and all of that, but it's what comes after that which causes me quite a bit of anxiety ....a trivial thing like temporary adjustments! Have I done it? Have I remembered to stop or start care? ... The temporary adjustment is purely administrative but it bothers me whether I've done it or not.

In the teams researched (Postle, 1999), the care managers initially were hopeful that a new computer system which was being introduced would reduce the amount of form filling thus alleviating the pressure caused by this and freeing them up to spend more time on direct work with people. The IT system, however, had a number of problems:

1.   It was cumbersome, using time which could be spent more beneficially on direct work with service users. As the following interview extract describes, the computer system, which in its early days was extremely slow (taking up to six minutes to clear each screen), had the drawback that until it had processed the assessment and care plan, and these had been authorised by the team manager and returned to the care manager, the contract for care could not be issued to the care agency:

It's not professional enough for me and I find that quite frustrating ... I've got people I should be going to visit and I can't get out and visit them because the priorities are to get the orders out. To get the orders out I've got to put the assessment on, put the order on, get it through the system, get it through vetting, get it through to be authorised and get it back into the print queue and get it back to be signed by the manager and then by myself and then out to the provider and, because I need that service, I've got to stay in here and get that out ... the whole care management process is actually being held up by the computer system

It appeared that the computerised assessment had been designed primarily to meet managerial needs for budgetary control and accountability. These are essential functions but clearly necessitate different approaches from those that would assist in assessing people's needs. This fits with the market ethos where clearly there is a need for expenditure controls, but it is mismatched with an assessment process that should focus on a person's view of their situation and their needs.

2.   It resulted in reductionist recording, which was not seen as being capable of recording people's needs accurately. The following were typical comments, which indicated staff's realisation that using IT assessment proformas circumscribed how they structured their assessments:

You become like the DSS officer where you tick the boxes ... you tick the boxes and you do the sums and you're not looking, you're not doing social work and that's terrible.

Doing the assessments on the computer just doesn't quite work. There are these 'pick boxes' you fill in and, although there's a bit where you can put free text, you need to do the 'picks' because they come up at the bottom, with 'needs identified', not with the text. So the 'needs identified' are the last bit on the assessment and you identify them and they are never quite right or exactly what I would say.

3.   Using this design of IT form was incompatible with good practice. Staff on a training course were told that they could use a printout from the IT form as a guide to collecting information because: *How you collect the information is down to you and your professional judgement.* Later, the trainer emphasised the importance of gathering and recording all the information the IT form required and advised staff to *Start thinking under headings.* Thus, in using the computerised assessment forms, staff were being advised to carry out a paradoxical injunction. They were to use professional skills and judgement in carrying out an assessment, but to ensure that their assessment was circumscribed, and thereby constrained, by the headings on the IT form.

Attempting to formalise and bureaucratise care management procedures is an application of what Blaug describes as *instrumental* reason. This is concerned with control and efficiency, ensuring that tasks are performed in a uniform way and hence well-suited to market transactions. Blaug compares this with *communicative* reason, concerned with interaction and emotion, (Blaug, 1995, p. 426). He further comments that such concentration on procedures can tend to help bad social workers and hinder good ones. Most care managers were experiencing a de-skilling of their role in terms of their reduced emotional labour and increased bureaucratic tasks. This was happening in a way that appears to be symptomatic of the wider process of casualisation and de-skilling (Simiç, 1995) and, indeed, of the commercialisation and commodification of emotional labour (Gorman, 2000b). It becomes clear that the concern expressed by some care management staff that their work could be done by unqualified staff is realistic.

Furthermore, the use of reductionist IT assessment procedures risks rejecting any notion of an 'exchange' model of assessment, which Smale *et al.*, (1993) describe as giving scope for a sharing of information between client and worker, and hence relying on the client's expertise in their situation. They contrast this with a 'questioning' model, which they demonstrate as one in which the worker, as 'expert', holds all the information and expertise. The notion of thinking under headings where these are restricted and prescribed by forms or computer systems epitomises a 'procedural' model, derived from the questioning model, and used to 'fit' clients to agency criteria or services (Smale *et al.*, 1993). Procedural and questioning models, which are reliant on agencies' or professionals' agendas, can never be empowering, as can be deduced from our discussion of empowerment in Chapter 5.

The care managers appeared to use information technology because it was available, regardless of its suitability for the task. It was as if failure to use it would be seen as a retrogressive step (Loader, 1998). It is questionable whether an IT system, while apparently purporting to be capable of enabling care managers to perform the task of assessment, is a simulacrum of the assessment itself. It appears to represent an assessment, while having none of its interactive, tacit, non-linear capacity and is, in fact, serving a different purpose from what it ostensibly appears to do.

What care managers do
- Paperwork generated by the operation of a market for care;
- Paperwork generated by restricted financial resources;
- Use IT programmes that are unsuitable for the assessment task; and
- Have limited time to spend in contact with people with whom they work.

(Webb *et al.*, 1998; Gorman, 1999b; Postle, 1999)

Care management – any care?

When considering the changed role of social workers to care managers earlier in this chapter we discussed the concerns that the potential for the appropriate use of therapeutic skills was reduced by the introduction of an increasing number of bureaucratic tasks. The use of self, however described, is recognised widely as an important and integral part of social work (Stevenson and Parsloe, 1993; Sheppard, 1995; Howe, 1996; Payne, 1996; England, 1998). The care work or 'emotional labour' that staff do lacks a language to describe it adequately (Camilleri, 1996), and care managers used a variety of terms such as '*client-centred stuff*', '*counselling*', '*listening*' and '*spending time*' to explain how they formed and worked within a relationship with people with whom they worked. There is a problem with the lack of descriptive words for this care work, or the use of words borrowed from the language of counselling or psychotherapy, yet lacking their concomitant meaning. It means that social work has left itself open for other terminology, particularly the managerialist discourse, to define its task. The terminology, and thereby the task, can appear meaningless to people outside social work and easily be denigrated by people, including those within the profession, who negate its integral nature in the care management task. This is exemplified in the following comment made by a team manager:

> *There just isn't the time for them to be giving of themselves in the way that they were and while that may be very nice for the client, and it may be very nice for them in terms of job satisfaction, it's not very good for the fifty people who are still waiting for someone to step through their door ... I'm not putting down the counselling, but it's got to be seen as something apart from what we do ... we should actually be purchasing counselling skills, buying them in from a secondary provider*

The discourse about care is problematic and paradoxical in nature. This is highlighted by Fox's helpful distinction between the nature of care referred to above and discussed by Camilleri, and care as 'vigil' or surveillance allied to the direct or indirect regulation of those people with whom care managers work (Fox, 1995). The feminised nature of care, in the sense of caring 'for', can be seen as derived from that which defines women's roles as 'natural' care-givers and therefore as being inherent in the feminised roles of people of either sex who carry out the caring task. As such, it is all too easy not to see this as 'work' but as something done as a matter of course and thereby rendered 'invisible' (Pithouse, 1987, Camilleri, 1996). However, Camilleri describes the emotional labour as not simply an addition to the work but rather as the 'real' work which:

> *Involves a heavy personal interaction and commitment. Engaging the client in terms of its rhetoric is more than just 'face to face work', it implies getting **inside** the person, understanding their feelings and emotions and using these to make sense of who they are and how they came to be here, that is, to be in need of social work help* (Camilleri, 1996, p. 84)

Again, it is important to note that this definition of 'real' work is contentious and would be contested by, for example, a Marxist critique of social work, placing greater emphasis on the importance of promoting social change (Sheppard, 1995; Jones, 1998). These differing discourses may not be as discrete and mutually exclusive as at first seems apparent. However, in discussing the care managers' comments about their work, their discourse is seen as being allied more closely to the description given by Camilleri. Gorman links Hochschild's sociological thesis in *The Managed Heart* (Hochschild, 1983) explicitly to research into care managers' work in terms of the commercialisation of human feeling and the corresponding cost to those workers of acting like emotional robots. The regulated nature of their work is seen as a result of increased managerialist control and loss of autonomy (Gorman, 2000b). Hence, as this care manager commented, care managers saw the real work of forming a relationship with clients as being core to their work and now being eroded by the time spent on bureaucracy and a fast turnover of work:

The quality of the relationship with the client seems to have changed... There's always been administration in social work... However, the paperwork and the bureaucracy was, compared to now, minimal... You had more time to see clients... [Now] you feel more remote from the client because you're whizzing in and you're setting up care and you're out and then you review again in three months and you don't build up those layers of knowledge about that person ... In the past, you could use yourself as a resource a bit more in providing that time or that listening ear, or if somebody was bereaved or whatever, it was quite appropriate to spend the time with the client, listening and counselling, not in a formal way ... now it's much more identifying the need and then actually contracting in a service.

A comment from another care manager provides an example of how an older person's concerns may well extend beyond the immediate need to resolve physical problems:

There's no services available to tap into that can buy trust ... Older people have fears about mortality starting to come to the surface that might not have been the case a few years earlier ... they need time to talk about these sorts of issues. Last week I was talking to a lady of 82 and she said, 'Are you frightened of dying?' That came from her, quite unsolicited.

The problems which older people face are as complex as those of any other group of people and are often compounded by a health component, cumulative loss and a need for strong advocacy (Marshall, 1989). It can be very helpful for older people and for people caring for them to have the opportunity to talk with a care manager who carries out emotional labour. This can help the older person to air their feelings and reach often difficult and painful decisions, rather than solely performing a bureaucratic task with them(Simiç, 1997).

Pressures of time and the changed nature of their work were squeezing out time for care managers to undertake essential care work and forcing them to adopt a much more cursory approach. Care work was becoming seen as something which could no longer be afforded or could, in some way, be short-circuited. For example, one of the training staff on an in-house training course advised staff that they should tell people to *'Tell me the problem sooner'* to avoid people telling them something really important right at the end of a visit or after several visits. This advice, intended to help the students to reduce their time pressures, relies on a bureaucratic, linear and procedural approach to the work in which the worker can fit the person to her/his schedule. It contrasts with notions of working at the person's pace and using tacit knowledge and reflection (Schön, 1991, Eraut, 1994) to enable and empower them to participate on a more equal basis in the assessment process. An alternative approach to that suggested by the trainer can be found in Biestek's work and appears closer to the caring nature of the work which the care managers were saying that they now found it difficult to do:

> *The function of the caseworker is principally to create an environment in which the client will be comfortable in giving expression to his feelings. The skill to create this environment is much more important than the skill of asking stimulating questions. In fact, the latter skill will be ineffective without the permissive atmosphere.* (Biestek, 1961, p. 40)

Despite constraints of time and the volume of paperwork, most care managers were attempting to do the skilled care work (Gorman, 1999b; Postle, 1999). Visits often revealed use of practice skills which indicated that, far from becoming de-skilled, most care managers demonstrated considerable skills in their purposeful use of themselves. Here is an example of this (pseudonyms have been used):

> *Charlie visited Mr Arthur aged 92, recently widowed, who was in hospital with varicose vein problems and pneumonia. It was a very complex situation in which Mr Arthur's family were refusing to allow him to be discharged back to a residential home, while the hospital were pressing for discharge. Legal advisers were involved on all sides. Charlie began his visit with a conversation with the consultant about the family's latest legal moves and what reports would be needed to 'cover' themselves if Mr Arthur's discharge went ahead. Charlie then went to see Mr Arthur, who told him that he was rather muddled about where his wife was. Sitting close to him, taking his hand and maintaining eye contact, Charlie*

explained, very gently, that it was hard for Mr Arthur to remember things, and that his wife had died. He remained attentive to Mr Arthur, reassuring him, before beginning to broach the subject of his move out of hospital.

What became apparent from such observations was that many care managers were, as the observation shows, still using skills which they associated with social work rather than care management practice, despite the concentration on bureaucratic, routinised care management tasks. Charlie's skill in dealing with Mr Arthur's question about his wife's whereabouts demonstrated his ability to understand both Mr Arthur's confusion at not realising his wife had died, and his potential for becoming upset and embarrassed when reminded of this. Also, he was able to put aside the considerable legal and administrative problems despite their disruptive potential and, instead, engage with Mr Arthur's concerns, staying with these until it was clear that, at least for the time being, Mr Arthur had understood.

Care managers, however, frequently commented on their loss of opportunity to use themselves skilfully in their work, feeling that such work was being squeezed out by increased bureaucracy. As one care manager indicated, they already regarded their use of themselves as '*undercover*' work. This interview extract indicates their views:

There seemed to be a lot more time to go out and spend time with people, listening to what's happening and then feeding it back. We even had time for listening as in, i.e. counselling. I don't tend to use the word 'counselling' because it's not a qualification I have, but I have listening skills ... The care component of care management seems to be slipping as you don't have time to spend with the client with all the other responsibilities as well.

It would be simplistic and incorrect to infer from care managers' comments that they thought there was a 'golden age' of social work in which staff spent time working on therapeutic relationships with their clients, did little if any paperwork, and yet kept paperwork up to date. However, as we have noted, care management has been characterised by apparent loss of time spent on direct contact work with people, in which some social workers felt that they were able to use therapeutic or counselling skills, and which could be said to constitute 'care'. This loss could also be seen as contributing to a change in the core relationship in which social workers engaged and worked with their clients. Such a fundamental change in the work, from direct work with potential for therapeutic input to considerably increased bureaucracy, leads to a questioning of the future role of social work itself (Simiç, 1995; Hadley and Clough, 1996).

Care management – any management?

The market for care has resulted in staff concentrating their efforts on managing individual packages of care. Care managers tended to work in individualised ways with people, looking at individual solutions to individual needs, rather than considering the broader picture of what could benefit a community and, in turn, the individual. The following interview extract, describing work with an elderly couple who were both in poor health, exemplifies this:

> *The scenario that I'm working with at the moment, which I particularly find quite ludicrous ... a couple would like to be picked up by minibus to go to their social club. The bus passes their door and there are two spaces on it ... Since the voluntary driver scheme stopped and it's been taken over by a care agency, anybody who wants to use that now ... needs to be screened and needs to be category 1. So this bus goes past their door and they're left to walk up the road, up a very steep hill.*

The care manager's description of the situation as '*ludicrous*' highlights the lack of opportunities for collective work with colleagues and other agencies which could obviate situations like this and provide preventative services (Clark *et al.*, 1998; Lewis *et al.*, 1999). Operating a market for care in conditions of restricted resources exacerbated the budgetary and, in turn, procedurally-driven natures of the work.

The flexibility to work in different ways was constrained by the procedural and individual nature of the work, emphasised by the statement that each person *needs to be screened and needs to be category 1*. Most care managers spoke of feeling too ground down by and consumed with routine work to think creatively and to look for other solutions which drew upon community networks, although they knew that preventative approaches would probably save time and be more beneficial for people (Gorman, 1999b; Postle, 1999). This lack of any collective response, moving beyond an individualised approach, together with short-termism, led to the false economy of ignoring all aspects of preventative work, as epitomised by this care manager's comments:

> *If someone's not clearly Category 1 but there are problems you can foresee, like two months, three months down the road, there's gonna be a significant problem, the feeling still seems to be, 'Well, no. Don't do anything now. Deal with the crisis three months down the road.'*

Staff efforts were targeted increasingly on very frail people, which, as this care manager explains, was a very short-sighted approach:

The nature of the work is such that, because there are more frail people able to be maintained in the community, the goalposts have shifted to the frail dependant ... Because the resources are limited, care must be focused almost exclusively to people who are Category 1 ... Obviously there are situations where a bit of care is going to sort of help further reduction, and so sometimes people can be a bit Category 2ish, if you like, but it's done on the basis of, as the saying goes, 'risk to the public purse'. That little bit now would help prevent deterioration.

This focus of the work on individualised packages of care for those people who are considered to be most in need, with need determined largely by degree of risk, is management of crisis not management of care. As we shall discuss further in Chapter 4, care managers operate in a prevailing climate of risk, reflecting the heightened sense of risk in the contemporary society in which they work (Giddens, 1991; Beck, 1992). This is a society concerned with the actuarial calculation of risk and its reduction/elimination, and yet one in which the new risks become increasingly difficult to manage (Giddens, 1991; Parton, 1996b; Ginsburg, 1998). Much care management work, particularly assessment, focuses on the extent to which someone is at risk and, indeed, this governs the 'eligibility criteria' for a service (Harding, 1997). At the same time many staff perceived a considerable risk of, at the least, complaints and, at worst, litigation against themselves or their Local Authorities, and their work was increasingly circumscribed by concerns about risks related to health and safety. Concurrently, however, the speed of work throughput did not give care managers time to evaluate and monitor risk properly, or spend time with people or their carers working on ways to reduce it. The sense of chaos experienced by care managers was compounded by a shift of focus of major conflicts and contradictions away from all staff in management positions, whose time is now taken up with strategic planning, budgetary monitoring and so on, towards front-line staff (Clarke, 1998). This is apparent in many of the boundary disputes which arise between health and social services personnel at front-line level, such as those concerning whether Health or Social Services should pay for care provision.

This individualised form of social work is doomed by its failure to see the broader picture of people's lives. For social work to survive it will need to recognise and explore new ways of working that will enable staff to lift their heads from the purely narrow focus of individualised work to address the social situations of the people with whom they work (Jordan, 2000; Smale *et al.*, 2000). Although this will require different ways of working at organisational and individual staff member level and across and between organisations and individual professionals, those who advocate such different approaches all agree that they are reliant on core social work skills and values (Payne, 2000; Smale *et al.*, 2000). Where innovators have responded to the challenge of operating in ways which keep in focus the societal context, the community and the individual, the beneficial results for people have been considerable (Holman, 2000; Lewis and Milne, 2000).

What needs to change?

- Re-evaluation of the operation of an extensive market for care;
- Re-evaluation of core social work skills and their application within the care management task;
- Approaches to work which maintain a balance of individual, community and societal needs rather than focusing solely on the individual;
- Organisational structures which allow for networking and are less dominated by managerialist approaches; and
- A training agenda incorporating continuing professional development.

Chapter 4
Decision-making about community care services
– dithering as an art form?

In previous chapters we have discussed factors that have influenced the development of community care and its interpretation through the rationing of community care services by social services departments and health trusts. Key factors in the current climate of decision making about who gets a service and the type of input they receive are:

- the influence of the market in welfare;
- value for money;
- cost containment;
- audit of social services activities;
- the effectiveness of inter-agency work (for example, service commissioning);
- a lack of community development and preventive work;
- continued dependence on family and informal carers;
- the values of individual care managers;
- changing professional roles; and
- risk and defensive practice.

The societal context is important to decision-making, as are legal requirements and agency constraints and conditions. Another key factor is the decision-maker's individual perspective on the merits of a particular case. This chapter will consider operational and personal issues affecting those who make decisions and those who are on the receiving end – the users of services and their carers.

Care management is the administrative and operational envelope in which decision-making activity related to the assessment and provisions of community care services continues to be realised. The context of the care manager's role and the role of the care manager can be understood by visualising the care manager at the intersection between 'top down' and 'bottom up' pressures. The context is the rationing of resources and devolution of responsibility, yet maintaining centralised control. There is potential for conflict from a range of sources, with the care manager being vulnerable to sinking under the weight of responsibility, legal challenge, and agency and service-user expectations. The care manager is at the centre of a range of conflicting imperatives (Gorman, 1999b).

The role of the care manager is a central theme of this book, as has been discussed in previous chapters. The care manager operates in a climate of role conflict and ambiguity, and it is in this climate that care management as the practical expression of care in the community is experienced by many users of services. Most of the tensions experienced by care managers relate to expectations about how they operate. The systems in which care managers operate have dominated their activity. Work, which was considered to be 'social' work before the community care reforms of the 1990s, has 'taken a back seat'. Areas of work with a focus on people such as therapeutic intervention and community development, although they are very different in their origins and philosophies, share a commonality of a preventive ethos. Trying to prevent breakdown, whether it be of an individual or within and part of a community, used to be accepted as part of the Local Authority Social Services' role. Most social workers who were also assessors for community care services would have preventive project work as part of their caseload. This reality was changed by the manner in which care management was implemented.

Care management, with its inherent ambiguities and tensions, is the context at the start of the twenty-first century in which care managers have to make decisions about who gets community care services. Evidence of conflict and ambiguity in the care manager's role is drawn from empirical research (Gorman, 1999b; Postle, 2002) and is illustrated below.

Figure 4.1   **The roles of the care managers**

THE ROLES OF THE CARE MANAGER

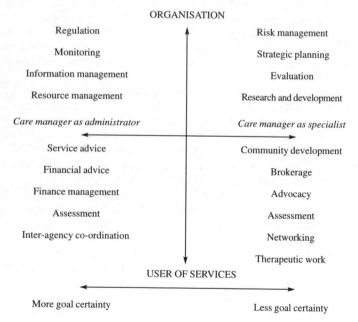

Role conflict and ambiguity

COMPLEXITY OF SYSTEMS WORK   COMPLEXITY OF PROFESSIONAL WORK

ORGANISATION

Regulation	Risk management
Monitoring	Strategic planning
Information management	Evaluation
Resource management	Research and development
Care manager as administrator	*Care manager as specialist*
Service advice	Community development
Financial advice	Brokerage
Finance management	Advocacy
Assessment	Assessment
Inter-agency co-ordination	Networking
	Therapeutic work

USER OF SERVICES

More goal certainty   Less goal certainty

Gorman, 1999b

44

The vertical axis represents a focus on the organisation (usually the Social Services Department) delivering care management, and contrasts this with a focus on the user of services. The horizontal axis represents the role of the care manager as a potential continuum from administrator to specialist professional. Each segment of the diagram represents the focus of care management activity dependent upon the prevailing forces. In essence the diagram shows role conflict and ambiguity emanating from difference between activity that has an organisational and systems focus and work that has a professional focus.

It is within this context that the care manager has to make decisions. A number of dilemmas arise that bring into question the nature of decision-making and our expectations about accountability – who is responsible for what?

This begs three important questions that relate to decision-making in community care:

- Is it possible to be an autonomous professional?
- Is it possible to be an empowered and independent recipient of services?
- Is it possible genuinely to advocate for someone when you have influence over the resources that they might receive?

One contextual factor that is relevant to service outcomes is the nature and extent of inter-professional work, and how far agencies are able to work together during the decision-making process.

Working inter-professionally: does it lead to better decisions for service users?

People who have taken part in team exercises will be aware of old adages that say, 'two heads are better than one' and 'the whole is greater than the sum of the parts' but they will also be aware of the saying 'too many cooks spoil the broth'. There is no doubt that good inter-disciplinary teamwork can be the best solution to providing holistic care for individuals. Much depends on the membership of the team, the way that decisions are made within such a team, and whether the users of services and their carers are involved in decision-making about the quality of their lives (Payne, 2000).

Care managers have been concerned about how working in collaboration with other professionals can lead to conflict:

I think collaboration is very difficult and I notice that we have a tendency to avoid it, to be honest, because of the difficulties, for example, what we are supposed to do is send off assessment forms to different people who have contact with the client for them to send back. Nine out of ten times I do it myself. Nine out of ten GPs won't send the form back anyway; they don't see it as their job.

There is a gulf between them and us despite joint strategies and so-called joint training. In practical terms, we have to tell them what to do. There are some exceptions to that – some good staff around who will get one of the assessment forms and do a really good job of it, but very often they go off and you never see them again, they rarely come back, so you cut corners and do it yourself.

I do think that we need skills to collaborate, to work well with other professionals, but some people do not want to do that, don't find that a useful way of working. They want to do brief assessments for straightforward tasks that are clearly defined by procedures and criteria ... they want to make brief relationships with people on that level and with that task. But I am not really interested in doing quick in/out assessments.

There are often differences of approach to the work, with social work trained care managers thinking that nursing and medical colleagues don't consult the client enough: *Occasionally there are various conflicts – maybe the situation arises where you think what are the person's needs here – but they forget to ask the person.*

It may be that conflict is inevitable when agencies and individuals try to work in collaboration with one another. Indeed, it is possible to say that conflict is part of collaboration in community care, and needs to be recognised as part of the process (Gorman, 2000b). At the same time there is evidence from our research (Gorman, 1999b, Postle, 1999) that, for example, care managers who work in rural areas with older people do work successfully together with community nursing staff because there is a sense of mutual dependency. Similarly, there were many comments about successful collaborative working practices in community mental health teams, where conflict between different 'professionals' was rare. One care manager commented that: *Spats don't happen so often now; we've developed very good policies and procedures and ways of doing things that work so we're not in conflict any longer.*

Collaboration with private care agencies is a significant change in the social work role. The impact of the private sector has changed the way that care managers make decisions about service provision. The creation and growth of the market in health and social care has caused a radical change in work within health and social care agencies. Many Social Services Departments buy in care, although in the early days of the community care reforms many authorities had maintained a large amount of in-house provision. For some care managers, good working relationships with private providers is a necessity, with collaborative skills centring on the transaction of care;

I maintain good working relationships with three of them, what I also like to do is use local ones. I can actually go up there with the purchase orders and the variation orders and sit down with them. We have a good working relationship and we can discuss what is best for the client.

As was discussed in Chapter 3, this approach is, however, anathema to others working in the same agency who think that management espoused the private-sector care agencies when they could have invested in public service agencies:

> *I think another problem with our management is that they shift with the fashion – when we started they were saying be adventurous, spend the money and using all the terms of the free market, then come September they say cut down, they just react to crises.*

Furthermore, staff felt that they had to make a decision about which agency to use. Care managers spoke about the variability in the standards of services, which offset the advantages of using a wider variety of service providers. The following two extracts from interviews exemplify this:

> *Some agencies, they slip. Their quality standards drop and then you're on edge.*

> [Agencies] *crop up all over the place ... one agency will come to our attention and we'll get good reports and we'll start using it. It seems like they've got this initial period when they are really helpful. We bombard them with work because they are doing well and they don't seem to want to refuse work, naturally, and they accept things when they really can't do it, and they'll be squeezing other clients and cutting corners. We'll use that agency for six months and then another agency's popped up willing to do things ... we'll move on.*

The variability of care agencies raised a number of issues including a lot of care managers' time being taken up in dealing with the problems arising from variability of service, such as carers failing to arrive. There was a lack of formal mechanisms for care managers to judge the standards of care provided by agencies, thereby placing service users at risk (Postle, 1999).

Issues related to the management of resources are at the nub of decision-making about community care services. There have been many legal challenges to decision-making by social services departments about the provision of services and the interpretation of the duties and powers of local authorities. The key legal decision in the Barry case (*R* v. *Gloucestershire County Council ex parte Barry* (1997)) was that local authorities could take resources into account when deciding on the provision of service even though they had a duty to provide. This decision has to be interpreted in the light of eligibility criteria decided by local authorities at Social Services Committee level. What is clear is that decision-makers must have a sound knowledge of current law relating to health and social care, and be able to work within it (Chand *et al.*, 2001).

Decision-making in care management – does it matter who your care manager is?

An interesting observation from research (Gorman, 1999b) is that users of services may be unaware of the significance of who the care manager is and how they represent users' cases when resources are allocated. There is a view expressed by care managers that users don't realise how important it is for them who their care managers are; there is concern about the internal battles they have to engage in to get services resources for their clients, so a client with a 'pushy' care manager may end up with more services. Underlying this feeling is the prime role of the social worker as an advocate for the client. This is a difficult role to play when the social worker is also the gatekeeper of resources, yet it is a role that traditionally has been accepted as part of social work theory, training and practice. For many the role of advocate has substantial meaning, while for others it has become something of a myth. Standing up for clients' rights may take the form of conflict with a range of other professionals:

> *I act as advocate; it's one of those things where again I think management doesn't see it as a high priority. I'm thinking in terms of the DSS ... we should be ... again it's pressure on time.*

> *The skill is working with people, it's advocating on their behalf, it's advocating to get them benefits, or whatever, that they deserve.*

> *The state has never liked us as advocates, like most of us I have had my share of run-ins with Social Security and Housing.*

The myth factor in the role of the advocate in social work expressed by Johnson (1972) is tied up with various interpretations of the meaning of the term. Some care managers are clear that they cannot really act as advocate when they are gatekeepers of resources, and they take the view that clients are better off having independent advocates.

> *It's very difficult to be both because if you are an assessor and a care manager you are a purchaser – aren't you? – so you can't. Although you feel that you want to be an advocate because the old social work is being an advocate for somebody – I think that is where the struggle lies.*

This quotation endorses the view that social workers did work as advocates in the 'golden age' of social work. This perspective is open to challenge as a myth, however. Some care managers may believe that they are acting as advocates when they are assessing and creating care packages, yet there is a subtle difference here between wanting the best for the client and actually acting as advocate on his/her behalf. Rather than advocacy, some care managers appear to be acting as mediators between the various actors, yet they may find it hard to exercise a mediator's crucial impartiality, thus making the task a virtual impossibility (Postle and Ford, 2000). Indeed, acting as a mediator rather than as an advocate may not always be in the person's best interests where, for example, there are clear power imbalances. Nonetheless, relationship-building is seen to be crucially important to some social workers acting as care managers. One care manager explains:

> *My perception (of the care manager role) is that the key to it is in the relationship and that applies now as much as ever it did. I think it is back to the old social work principles of building a relationship, that people are all very different, that they can be difficult, that conflict is always around and it isn't just a job of putting care packages in. What is important is dealing with conflict, being sensitive, because very often users of services are going through a time of change and loss.*

Decision-making and acting as the 'Street Level Bureaucrats' – a powerful role for care managers?

The downgrading of professional tasks and a focus on outcomes rather than the processes of care has been a stressful and disheartening experience for many care managers, especially those who were fieldworkers before the move to care management, and became care managers working primarily with elderly people. The opportunity to improvise, and to use practice wisdom to the best advantage is often, but not invariably, lost. There appear to be three sets of reactions at play: accommodation, resistance and a response to day-to-day pressure that may not necessarily be in the best interests of the users of the service. In *Street Level Bureaucracy* Lipsky (1980) recounts similar dilemmas of the individuals in the public service. There is a rearguard action of social worker/care managers re-owning social work skills (for example, honing assessment skills) and seeing new opportunities, such as a significant role in the commissioning of services. The 'going the extra mile' is not necessarily viewed as something that is rewarded by the employer organisations, who are seen by some as reacting to the fashion, paying more attention to appearance rather than reality. The response of some care managers is consciously to play the system, or at least make the system work for them. They have had to learn fast in a welfare world that now includes the private sector. These reactions range from exaggerating a client's needs in order to get appropriate funding for care, to being less than precise about the completion of workload monitoring audits, ignoring administrative demands and taking more time with clients than would meet managerial approval. A notion of 'social worker charisma' can arise, bordering on bravado at being able to survive the system:

I am not an administrator, I don't have that, and I've never developed those skills. I'm accused of being an anarchist, which is probably fairly true.

If I go and see a client I'll stop and have a cup of tea with them, have a chat with them, you know. I mean, a manager might see that as a complete waste of time but I don't.

If you are getting pressure to do more paperwork or more procedures which you can't see the point of but which actually prevent you from client contact you tend to think – oh sod it, I'll do the visits and sort the rest out later.

Such reactions can be interpreted as part of the commodification of emotion in labour that is accomplished through the transmutation of elements of emotion as a public rather than a private act, the directors of the act being not the individuals themselves but the managers, with 'feeling rules' being spelt out in rule books so that autonomy over the use of emotion is restricted (Gorman, 2000b). There is some evidence of passion in performance, of suffering in the carrying out of organisational roles and some organisational nostalgia. Care managers who are in the purchasing role are conscious of the risk of criticism, or at worst, complaints:

In order to maintain my independence – and I'd say that every care manager has a different strategy – if it's left to me I keep a spread of three care agencies. I thought three was a good number – I can't be accused of taking back-handers.

There are two basic things – don't go over budget and don't get a complaint against yourself.

I have had to learn to work with the private sector. Often there is a home with a vacancy and they will ring us up as individuals. I want to tell them that's your problem, you are a private business; don't lean on me. I have to be polite. This requires conflict management – covering your back. When community care was first mooted I said then that we would be open to this sort of abuse, to allegations etc.

It is in this welfare climate that decisions are made daily about the allocation of scarce community care resources. It is useful to consider some examples of decision-making dilemmas.

Should a care manager decide to offer care that matches a user's preference, or a service that the agency considers meets the user's basic needs?
Take the situation of Susie, who has learning disabilities. She wants to go to the Cedars day-care facility because she can swim there. She finds that swimming helps her to relax and keep mobile. However, the nearest day-care facility does not have a swimming pool. There is also some difference in cost. The care manager has been told by a senior manager to offer the nearer day-care facility.

Should a care manager talk up a client's case so that eligibility criteria are met? When is someone frail enough to trigger a service?
Take this example: Mrs Jones is 84 and she lives alone, has occasional dizzy spells and is arthritic. She is getting very upset because her net curtains need washing and she needs some help with the housework. Her neighbours think that she is 'going a bit strange' and getting depressed and worked up about the state of her house.

Should a care manager continue to commission services that he/she knows are not really very good quality, but about which there have been no official complaints?
There have been a number of reports from the home care service that a lot of the meals provided by 'X Caterers' purchased by social services are not really meeting the dietary needs of ethnic minority elders. There have been occasions when unsuitable meals have been provided for vegetarian clients. It was also known that apples were ordered for people who had no teeth!

Should a care manager get involved in wider issues relating to care and protection that may involve the police?
Agnes, an elderly woman aged 90, has told her home care assistant that her son has been demanding money from her on a regular basis. However, a duty visit to the home reported that Agnes denied all knowledge of this. The home carer continues to report to her supervisor Agnes's distress after the son's visits.

Should a care manager keep open cases of older users when the operation of the case management system used in the office results in closing cases as soon as intervention is complete?
Jim, an older service user, has had alcohol problems and while he manages quite well he goes out at nights to the local pub and occasionally cannot find his way back home, eventually sleeping rough in the local park. He is not considered a complex case, but he does present the occasional risk to himself and others.

The dilemmas decscribed above relate to decisions that care managers have to make on a regular basis. The main elements for consideration in decision-making in this context can be isolated as:

- interpretations of risk and frailty;
- interpretations of the rights of users and carers;
- interpretations of need in a climate of rationed resources;
- interpretations of the duties and powers of local authorities in relation to eligibility criteria; and
- interpretations of the extent of continued professional support, that is, the social work role.

The role of the care manager is circumscribed by the domain of management in the sense that authority is dependent upon law and policy and the power vested in public servants. However there is an element of decision-making that relates to professional discretion and the personal values that the practitioner brings to the decision-making process (Gorman *et al.*, 1996). It has been recognised that the orientations of practitioners are significant in decisions made in social work (Stevenson and Parsloe, 1993). A variety of forces can affect decision-making outcomes, including the family background and early socialisation of officials, their education, the influences of religion and politics as well as the continuing changing values of society. Athough they are in a minority in our research, some care managers have seen advantages in the changes to care management. They consider that there is more potential flexibility in the choice of services and scope to get to know more about users' needs. The comments from one care manager illustrate this point:

Care management can be rewarding because we can buy services in, which is something we never had before, it is a wonderfully powerful thing ... a couple of years ago I could not get anything. One can have influence on the way money is spent... there is a certain amount of autonomy in spending up to a limited amount without referring back.

It would be interesting to speculate which elements have the greater influence in specific case decisions such as those outlined above. It could be argued that agencies constrain, if not erode, professional values, replacing them with technical and procedural decision-making practice. However, it may be that the 'community care revolution' has taken the lid off and exposed some of the processes involved in decisions about eligibility that had remained largely unchallenged because of the power of authority vested in the professional 'to make the right decisions'.

The application of the Human Rights Act 1998 should have an influence on decision-making about community care services. It is now more important than ever that decision-makers are clear about their reasons for making a decision, and that they record those reasons. It may be an opportunity for care managers to humanise systems that are often bewildering to the uninitiated. It may be impossible for those making decisions about who gets what service to be entirely 'neutral', but it may be possible to make appropriate decisions based on ethical principles derived from a reflective and critical study about one's own activity as a care manager. The evaluation of planned care should be part of the skills repertoire of care managers, but this needs to be a process geared to strategic policy, planning and training initiatives (Gorman, 2000c).

Accountability and the decision-making process

Care management and specifically assessment processes have developed predominantly as managerial systems concerned with the cost-effective administration of resources (Futter and Penhale, 1996; Lewis and Glennester, 1996). At the same time, the policy of promoting user choice and self-determination has been a theme of the community care reforms, potentially redefining the professional role in service delivery. This left care managers in something of a quandary in terms of the balance between their perception of their accountability to the organisation as a bureaucrat charged with a responsibility to manage resources (or at least be aware of the cost and limitations in services), and their perception of their professional accountability towards the client or user of the service. The ideas incorporated in the notion of user choice sit well with the ethics of social work, although such an ethical stance may be compromised by the notion of consumerism. The Department of Health did envisage that consumers of welfare could use an open and available complaints procedure and be encouraged to play an active part in the process of the management of their care (DOH, 1990). Yet choice for users has been exposed as a myth in the context of social services provision (Schorr, 1992), choice, in practice, being related strongly to what is available and a factor that relates to the possibility of social exclusion. By contrast, social inclusion could, for example, encompass the flexibility to purchase alternative therapies (Valios, 2001).

The role of care manager as advocate is compromised in a context of a purchaser/provider divide because, whereas professionals might focus on the needs of individual clients and seek out ways to maximise their opportunities for care, the care manager as purchaser and/or as provider may focus on the needs of populations or groups with an eye on cost containment.

The autonomy of the professional as care manager has been limited by the purchaser/provider split that allows other judgements of need to compete with or take precedence over professional judgements (Harrison and Pollitt, 1994). The concept of need central to the official versions of care management is contentious, and reflects the conflicts in theories of human need and the contexts in which they are applied (Doyal and Gough, 1991). Lewis and Glennester (1996) have concluded that the conflict between needs and resources implicit in the care manager role has been made explicit by the process of defining need in terms of a combination of risk, need and statutory responsibility. They consider that the rhetoric of needs-led services has resulted in a hierarchy of need that legitimises the failure to meet lower-level needs.

Let us consider this example:

Mrs B is an African Caribbean woman aged 80 who lives alone and has no immediate family living in this country. She has recently been discharged from hospital following a fall at her home. She is becoming increasingly frail because of arthritis, but she does not want to go into residential care. She can still manage some household tasks but has difficulty in lifting and carrying. She needs help with her cleaning and laundry, and gets very distressed when her living accommodation is not as clean as she would like it to be. Her friend who visits daily reports that Mrs B is getting increasingly depressed because she needs help in the house.

How would you help Mrs B if you were assessing her for community care services? Initially, the issue would be whether Mrs B meets the access or eligibility criteria following assessment. Even if she does meet the criteria, it may be that her situation is not considered to trigger the need for a service. This is a legally viable position and reflects the discretionary element of the decision-making process (Schwehr, 1999). The decision about the nature and type of service is potentially at the care manager's discretion, possibly confirmed by a team manager. We could not assume that the decision in this case would be the same in a different local authority.

For Lipsky (1980) criticism of the 'street level bureaucrats' who failed to deliver responsive and appropriate services to the community was explained by an analysis of the problems that social workers experienced in reconciling needs, resources and the ambiguous aims of the bureaucracy. He suggests that the exercise of professional discretion was problematic in a context where demand outstrips supply, recognising that the work orientations of public-sector bureaucrats determined a great deal of actual public policy as experienced by the users of services. He comments on the desire of 'street level bureaucrats' to maintain their discretionary capacity and being interested in processing work consistent with their own preferences and those agency policies that were so salient as to be backed up with agency sanction. 'Street level bureaucrats' may also use existing regulations and administrative provision to circumvent reforms that limit their discretion. The findings in our research (Gorman, 1999b; Postle, 1999) are consistent with Lipsky's themes, in the sense that care managers displayed a sense of alienation and the need for rearguard actions or personal strategies of action to confirm their professional identity and their personal standards about whether someone was deserving of their help. Lipsky identifies the high degree of uncertainty that characterises the role of the worker at the interface of user demand and managerial control characterised by the complexity of the subject matter (people), and the frequency or the rapidity with which decisions have to be made.

How care managers function within a bureaucracy may depend in part on how the individual worker manages the balance between their accountability to the client or user of the services and accountability to the welfare organisation as an agent of the state; an omnipresent dichotomy. As Mullaly (1993) points out, social workers are constrained in a variety of ways by various means: individual supervision, and a reward structure based on conformity to agency need rather than service-user need. As discussed in Chapter 3, heavy caseloads and computerisation all compound the problem. This is further exacerbated for care managers by the shift in worker time away from the client to the administrative processes necessary for the management of care: the increased monitoring of work activity coupled with an expectation that the care manager will co-ordinate the activities of others both within and outside the organisation.

Whereas, in social work, the rules governing accountability have often remained hidden, for the care manager the dilemma of *to whom* to be accountable becomes more intense. Pearson (1982) suggests that in social work the rules governing accountability are rarely explicit; there is scant acknowledgement of the public-knowledge component of a client's engagement with an agency, there is a problematisation process that centres on the client, and a lack of awareness that as the objects of large-scale organisation with bureaucratic features that they will be treated as ciphers within the administrative machinery.

What then, if anything, makes the work of care managers different from that of the social worker in relation to interpretations of accountability? It is possible to view the fragmentation of the care management process, the separation of simple from complex assessments, as a prescriptive process that is 'technicised' by the identification of need, the cost of services, and in the assessment and review of services. The Department of Health's seven stages of the care management process, underwritten by a range of proformas outlined in the government guidelines, emphasise the importance of procedures. Quality assurance runs alongside care management with a focus on the quality of the service provided by the care manager and the quality of the provision received by the user of service – the consumers. The accountability of the care manager could be sealed to the process of care management itself.

The notion of professional autonomy is bound up with a sense of accountability to the clients or users of services. This in turn relates to conceptions of professional values. England (1986) articulates the emotional difficulties that can be faced by social workers when they feel that their professional values have been compromised by the welfare bureaucracy that employs them.

Writing in 1986, England concludes that the organisation of social work poses problems of immense complexity, and this situation is compounded by a lack of clarity about the social work task so that neither the social worker nor the agency is clear about their role. Social work has never been differentiated in the agency from the routine provision of social services; indeed, the way in which social services organisations have evolved have been inimical to social work practice. Hadley and Clough (1996) make a similar comment in their more recent research into the impact of community care changes on the professional roles. A codified and bureaucratic response to need has dominated the construction of care management in the UK, with its emphasis on a bounded, needs-led service that has often masked realities of resource limitation. For care managers who were trained as social workers, this shift of emphasis has highlighted tensions that already existed (but were less explicit) in social work practice prior to care management implementation. It has been argued that the process of assessment, central to care management, enables social work to show its worth through the accomplishment of comprehensive and holistic assessments (Stevenson, 1995). Implicit within this notion is the reinforcement of social work skills in making relationships with clients, enabling them to manage their difficulties (Beresford and Trevillion, 1995; Payne, 1995; Brandon and Hawkes, 1998).

Yet care management has in the main been implemented with an emphasis on administrative and managerial systems. The focus has shifted away from quality time with clients to a notion of quality bound up with the monitoring of interventions, the categorisation of clients into eligible and non-eligible, and the rationing of resources. Social Services Departments would appear to have little or no interest in relationship building – a core element of the social work task. This dichotomy has taken on another twist in the debate between case management and care management and is related to the role of the care manager as an autonomous professional – which is perhaps a myth enhanced by professional training agencies, and higher education and awarding bodies.

Yet some improvements for individual users have been noted in research on care management (Hadley and Clough, 1996), although preventive work in general was identified as a potential casualty (Lewis *et al.*, 1995). At the same time, this reality that the nature of the work no longer encompasses a preventive element is resisted by workers in care management (Hadley and Clough, 1996), and this is borne out by the research findings (Gorman, 1999b). The notion that preventive work is part of past work reflects nostalgia for a golden age, which is a phenomenon that influences how present-day events are interpreted. This can be significant in an emotional gulf that separates the older organisational members from the younger ones, who may not have shared those experiences. Organisational nostalgia, with its emphasis on the emotional and the symbolic, can have the effect of vindicating a set of alternative values in organisations from those of profit, rationality, efficiency and domination (Fineman, 1993).

There is evidence that special projects, independent of existing bureaucracies and funded independently, enable an assessment of needs which can be transformed into an agreement between the client and the care manager about what might be done. Advocacy was a strong feature of the care management project with disabled people as described by Pilling (1992) and endorsed by Brandon and Hawkes (1998). The case manager in the project described by Pilling negotiated with representatives of the agencies providing the services, arguing the client's case. Their unattached status freed them to be able to complain and be forceful in a way that social workers conscious of hierarchy, authority policy and elected members could not (Dant and Gearing, 1993).

The notion of being an advocate for the client still remains part of the identity of many of the social workers working as care managers within Social Services Departments. Yet advocacy is a tricky concept, because it has a variety of interpretations. Brandon and Brandon (2002) discuss the various interpretations of the term, concluding that a key ingredient of such a warm and respectful process lies in the accomplishment of tasks defined by the client. The need to help the users of services, and to be responsive to the needs of those whom the professional helper perceives as being worthy of help, is tied up with the art of helping and notions of altruism that have a historical base in social work. They have formed a small part of the claims to professional status made by social workers and the organisations that represent them that has been codified in the British Association of Social Workers (BASW) Code of Ethics. This emotional labour, a responsiveness to other human beings in the context of work, is an interesting concept when applied to the role of the care manager, an occupation that has subsumed some of the elements of the social work role yet comprises a number of tasks and conventional responses to human dilemmas that requires the worker to behave in a regulated way. The circumscription of the role through the use of administrative forms and procedures, and the application of imposed eligibility criteria coupled with the lack of importance given to the development of personal relationships other than to define need, have all affected the emotional labour of the care manager, as discussed in Chapter 3.

Decision-making and the community?
But what has happened to community social work? One care manager from an inner-city area says:

> *As an automatic way of working it is less than it was ... it's really all gone now. I think people feel stressed doing their job – if you suggest that they should be doing something else (like community work) they say we can't do that — we don't have time.*

One of the legacies of the 'community care revolution' was the focus on a model of community care that emphasised the organisation of community care services through management systems rather than encouraging the community to make decisions about services that were needed. Individual care plans emphasised a fragmented approach to the delivery of care services. The NHS and Community Care Act 1990 was about assessing individual need and managing to meet those needs within limited budgets. As both Mayo and Popple (Mayo, 1994; Popple, 1995) explain, community care as it has been configured is not usually linked to community development strategies. It could be argued, however, that there are opportunities to link the Social Services agenda to local regeneration initiatives that have found more favour with the government in power at the time of writing. There are many projects that are funded through the Single Regeneration Budget and European funding that could pave the way for new forms of community work, or even community action to enable communities to increase their independence. Community regeneration has been developed by the current government through a public health agenda based on Health Improvement Zones (HIMPs) and Health Action Zones (HAZs). Stronger links could be made between Social Services Departments and other agencies within both the public and the private sectors. Joint funding could enable community partnerships to develop and flourish.

Care managers have to be aware that by exercising their powers of decision-making they can influence the promotion of independence for users. A more widespread use of the Direct Payments Act 1996 is one example. Bright and Drake (1999) report that user involvement in direct payments has been slow to get off the ground, especially with people with mental health problems and those with learning disabilities. Local authorities can impose an entry restriction – for example, people needing less than £80-worth of care a week are excluded. It is possible that care managers assess with this restriction in mind, despite evidence that direct payments are sometimes cheaper than service-based support (Hasler *et al.*, 1999).

Conclusion: decision-making and community care in transition

Difficult decisions have to be made by care managers about community care services in a climate of rationed resources. There may be several factors that enter the equation when a decision is made, and these include interpretations of law and policy, local demands and priorities, and the individual care manager's preferences.

One way of approaching the problems of decision-making in this context is for practitioners faced with such dilemmas to reflect on the process of what they are doing. Consideration of the following questions should help:

- Am I making a critique of my own practice?
- Have I engaged in a systematic process of decision-making that included evidence for the decision I have made?
- Have I taken into account an understanding of power relationships in the creation of a care compact that reflects users' and carers' wishes?

Berkowitz, in Ramon (1992), emphasises the importance of social workers' analysing what they do both in terms of the organisational structure and the culture in which they work. This message is a sound one in the context of care management activity, for greater transparency in decision-making is required when resources are limited. This imperative has been reinforced by the Human Rights Act 1998, which demands explanation in decision-making and accuracy in reporting reasons. The application of rules in the form of legitimate eligibility criteria should not be viewed as a set of chains that cause practitioners to sink under the weight of responsibility. Rules and regulations are necessary to assist in equitable decision-making, but they need to be applied in a climate of explicitness of intent and mutual respect. Care managers need to be imaginative about the possibilities of meeting assessed need.

Decision-making in care management, perhaps by its very nature, is dithering as an art form. It takes place in a climate of uncertainty and risk, and very often decisions have to be made in a context where there cannot be a 'right' decision. This is why it is imperative that confident and competent persons make those decisions, taking on board the wishes and rights of those who will experience the outcomes.

One clear question remains – does it have to be like this? It is likely that the tensions described above will remain, but the admittedly gloomy picture that emerges from some of our research findings is not the whole story. There were also expressions of hope and some positive activity aimed at making care management work for service users. One very practical example, discussed in this book and by previous commentators (Brandon, 1998), is the positive use of direct payments.

Brandon (1998) reminds us that the role of professionals is to give advice, but not to make decisions for others. This way of thinking requires social services departments to take the issues raised in this chapter on board in a genuine and purposeful way. Other key factors linked to this are the morale of staff and their need for continuing professional and personal development. Chapter 6 will raise issues relating to the workforce and the process of transforming community care.

Chapter 5
Empowerment

An overworked word or a meaningful concept?
Recently one of us was teaching a group of DipSW students when one of them commented:

'Empowerment' must be the most overworked word in social work. I feel sick whenever I hear it!

We have to admit that, when faced with student observation sheets which ask us to comment on how the student was 'empowering' during a visit or, when midway through marking a pile of student assignments we read:

I empowered Mrs Smith by contacting the housing department

We cannot help but agree with the student's view that 'empowerment' is an overworked word! It doesn't have to be like this, though! While acknowledging that empowerment is a term which has been reduced to jargon through over-use and lack of clarity, Croft and Beresford explain that,

For service users, empowerment means challenging their disempowerment, having more control over their lives, being able to influence others and bring about change (Croft and Beresford, 2000, p. 116).

People who have experienced paternalistic, patronising and clearly disempowering social work and/or community care provision (Morris, 1991; Oliver, 1996; Shakespeare, 2000) leave their readers in no doubt that this serves only to reinforce notions of dependency. As Shakespeare observes:

The institutionalisation of helping through community care often fails those who have a right to expect their needs to be met. Alongside the well-known failures of residential care (inflexible routine, lack of choice, dependence on others, lack of privacy) have to be set the failures of empowerment and participation which are clear from evaluations of community care. The current climate for many service users – older people, people with HIV/AIDS, disabled people and people with learning difficulties or mental health problems – is of minimal services and maximal dependency. (Shakespeare, 2000 p 57)

For older people, who have historically been marginalised by social services provision (Marshall, 1989; Hugman, 1994) and who may encounter simultaneous forms of discrimination, such as permutations of age plus gender, sexuality, 'race' and/or disability, issues of empowerment are particularly pertinent.

It is important to acknowledge that empowerment is a complex and contested term which, somewhat deceptively, is often used in a non-problematised way, as if its meaning was uncontested and it was an unquestioningly good concept. As Servian suggests, there is a danger that we assume we know what empowerment means (Servian, 1996). In reality, as his research with stakeholders in services for people with learning disabilities demonstrated, there is little agreement about its meaning. Further, empowerment can be paradoxical in that, in some situations, one person may feel empowered at the expense of another's perceived disempowerment (Servian, 1996). A recent example of this paradox can be found in Clark and Spafford's work about the extension of the direct payments scheme to older people. They found that, when carers used the scheme as a way to obtain more choice over their caring arrangements (such as by buying respite care), this resulted in a potential reduction in choice for the people for whom they cared (Clark and Spafford, 2001). As in examples given by Servian, this could be seen as empowering carers, but at the possible risk of disempowering people for whom they care.

Empowerment can be misunderstood and misused, as in the essay quoted at the beginning of this chapter, thus rendering it empty and meaningless, as implied by the student's comment. It can also be used in false notions of 'partnership' where power imbalances remain, or taken to mean a process of adaptation to, and acceptance of, powerlessness (Langan, 1998). In discussing *partnership*, Shardlow helpfully identifies its problematic nature. As we noted in Chapter 2, this is another term that can appear uncomplicated and has found its way into much policy guidance in a way which suggests consensus about its meaning. However, the term implies notions of equality and power balance which are not usually present in the relationships between social workers and service users (Shardlow, 2000). Shardlow suggests that this relationship is particularly unequal where social workers are involved in the protection of vulnerable people, or in statutorily defined work. We would add that the inequality inherent in the care manager's role as rationer of restricted resources also militates against notions of partnership.

Humphries highlights the inherent contradiction of working towards inclusion and empowerment within a societal context of anti-welfare consensus in which trends are towards social exclusion, polarisation and marginalisation (Humphries, 1996). While she locates the origins of these societal trends in the New Right policies of Thatcherite governments, critics of the New Left would see a continuation of these trends into current government policies (Jordan and Jordan, 2000).

There is a risk of becoming so bogged down in debates about the difficulty of defining empowerment that its meaning and importance for service users, highlighted at the start of this chapter, become lost. Because this is a complex area and yet one which is all too easily over-simplified, we have provided suggested further reading about empowerment at the end of this chapter. To summarise: the context in which we are using 'empowerment' involves a shift in the locus of control and monopoly of expertise from professionals to people using services. This shift needs to happen in ways that challenge inequality, oppression and discrimination in all their many forms (Smale *et al.*, 1993; Hugman, 1994; Braye and Preston-Shoot, 1995; Burke and Harrison, 1998; O'Brien and Penna, 1998). Drawing on Foucault's work, the understanding of empowerment underpinning the discussion throughout this chapter embodies the notion of power as relational and capable of generating resistance, not something fixed that can be given to or shared with another (Foucault, 1984). In this context, there is the potential for what Leonard describes as *collective resistance* against sites of struggle (Leonard, 1997, p. 169).

Notions of empowerment in care management
The rhetoric of empowerment runs throughout the community care reforms as the following extracts demonstrate:

> *Central government should look in detail at a range of options for encouraging individuals to take responsibility for planning their future needs* (Griffiths, 1988, p 22)

> *Promoting choice and independence underlies all the Government's proposals* (DOH, 1989, p. 4)

> *The rationale for this reorganisation is the empowerment of users and carers* (SSI and SWSG, 1991b, p. 7)

To date this rhetoric seems to have proved empty. Care management was influenced by a combination of consumerism, brokerage, service effectiveness, informal care, voluntary provision, social care planning and decentralised delivery (Levick, 1991). The lack of any definition of the role of care managers left Local Authorities free to interpret guidance, building on some existing good practice and on information from the pilot schemes researched by the Personal Social Services Research Unit (PSSRU) (Challis and Davies, 1986). Although these pilot studies were very influential as theoretical models, it is questionable how beneficial a model could be when, despite its appearance of innovation and good practice, it had not altered the dependency status of service users. In addition to replicability and preventative intervention, other issues were called into question by the adoption of care management models based on the pilot studies, not least the low wages and potential exploitation of (usually female) carers (Ungerson, 1993).

Overall, the outcome of policy based on the pilot studies suggests the metaphor of the production of a Morgan car. Such vehicles are lovingly hand-built to the customer's specifications over a number of months but, with an order waiting list of well over a year, they are only ever available for a tiny minority of drivers. Further, it can be argued that the goals of solely improving efficiency and targeting resources indicated by the results of the pilot studies may well not result in better outcomes for service users (Henwood, 1992).

Some models of care management, such as those which operated not-for-profit brokerage services, provided people with individual advice and linked them to services they chose (Huxley, 1993). These offered scope for user empowerment in which people could be experts on their own needs, thus emphasising their choice and independence (Smale *et al.*, 1993; Payne, 1995). This is particularly the case where some brokerage agencies' advisers have themselves had experience of being service users (Dowson, 1995). However, despite the emphasis on service-user involvement and choice noted above, hierarchies were perpetuated in the reforms and the avoidance of a clear brokerage model ensured that the power imbalance between professional and service user was not redressed. Service users may apparently have been given flexibility and choice, but none of the models gave them the money to exercise these fully (Hugman, 1991b). As we noted in Chapter 2, there have been subsequent attempts to redress this by the operation of the Direct Payments Act 1996, and research indicates that, if people using services are involved in direct payment schemes from the outset, these can prove to be empowering (Dawson, 2000). However, it is worrying to note that that Local Authorities may apply rigid and restrictive eligibility criteria to people wanting to use the direct payments scheme, thus retaining considerable control over its operation and perpetuating notions of dependency and lack of choice. Such rationing of resources can militate against the strategies for empowerment inherent in direct payments schemes (Clark and Spafford, 2001).

Throughout the implementation and development of community care policies, the least considered care manager role has been that of service users acting as their own care managers. The credibility of this approach, which indicates clear possibilities for user involvement and empowerment, is demonstrated in the case studies reported by Goss and Miller (Goss and Miller, 1995). These studies show care management work moving from a standpoint of 'them and us' to 'us and us' in a partnership based on a relationship of equality which recognises the equal, but different, expertise of users, carers and staff.

In writing about the community care reforms, Hugman warned that their inherent managerialist concerns could:

Perpetuate the existing view of work with this group [older people] as routine, prescribable, and ultimately of lower status, thereby reinforcing ageism (Hugman, 1994, p. 251).

Hence, while the language of the reforms appeared to be anti-discriminatory and empowering, the managerialist notion of the care manager operating as the interface between user and market highlights the market values inherent in the reforms. It signals a reductionist approach which, by its very nature, cannot hope to address discrimination (Hughes, 1995). Similarly, such managerialist approaches do nothing to redress power imbalances between staff and people who use community care services. As we have noted, notions of partnership, which can all too readily be misleading and vague in their understanding of equality, need to be unpacked carefully (Shardlow, 1999). Imbalances in equality need to be acknowledged and addressed to enable empowerment to take place (Brandon and Brandon, 1987).

Care management: empowering older people or exacerbating dependency?
The descriptions of care managers' visits to elderly people, given in this section, are taken from recent research (Postle, 1999) and serve to illustrate that, while some empowerment strategies were used, in many cases the care management process served to endorse, if not to exacerbate, dependency.

The following description of a care manager's visit to an elderly woman indicates the potential for ways of working which employ empowerment strategies:

Rosemary visited Mrs Lindford, a widow, aged 81. Mrs Lindford was in poor health, with diabetes, angina and infarcts. She was blind and both of her legs had been amputated. After being in hospital, following a stroke, she had gone to stay in a residential home. Assuming she would remain there, Mrs Lindford's family had cleared her flat and sold all her possessions without her agreement. She was desperately unhappy in the residential home, was losing weight and saying she wanted to return home. Mrs Lindford's family had recently stormed out of a review meeting, having refused to consider her return home and telling her, 'If you were a dog we'd have put you down!' In the face of this opposition, and with considerable concerns about Mrs Lindford's ability to cope, Rosemary none the less wanted to work with Mrs Lindford to assess whether a return home would be feasible. She took Mrs Lindford back to her empty flat, where the warden and a friend greeted her warmly. It was a slow process, with Rosemary giving Mrs Lindford a lot of time to look at her flat and to have tea with her friend and the warden. Rosemary listened attentively to what Mrs Lindford said and also noted her expression of delight when she was back in her, albeit bare, flat. She discussed the feasibility of Mrs Lindford's return with the warden and they outlined possible support networks. Mrs Lindford later returned home.

The pressures were considerable for Rosemary to rush a visit like the one described, or to take the line of least resistance and concur with Mrs Lindford's family's view that she would not be able to cope at home. However, by taking time and observing carefully, she was able to establish what Mrs Lindford wanted and what the warden felt was feasible. The cup of tea gave Mrs Lindford a chance to start to re-establish her support networks and make her own assessment about returning home. It gave Rosemary time to assess the extent of these networks, and Mrs Lindford's relationship with the warden, which would be crucial if she were to be able to return. An assessment focusing predominantly on risk, made after a brief visit, might have indicated that, with her poor health and her family's attitude (and their potential for complaint) Mrs Lindford would have been better left in the residential home, unhappy or not. But, this would have wrested all control from Mrs Lindford, leaving her disempowered and with what remained of her life controlled by others, on whom she would have had no choice but to be dependent.

By contrast, this description of a care manager's visit was more typical of ways of working that were becoming increasingly common:

Elaine visited Miss Allen, who was 83, lived alone and had been referred by the District Nurse who had described her as hard of hearing and very much at risk, but refusing services. During the visit Elaine focused most of her questions on risk and spent no time on finding out anything about Miss Allen's background and little about her interests. There were obvious risks in the house: an unguarded fire in a cluttered room, loose mats and steep stairs, but Miss Allen appeared to be fiercely independent and made it clear that she did not want help. Elaine told her that she would visit again in a couple of weeks. Elaine explained that, on this next visit, she would discuss Miss Allen's background and talk a bit more but, if she refused services, she would just have to record this fact and close the case. Elaine stated that she did not think this gave her time to get to know Miss Allen and that the focus was on risk.

Care management work takes place in a climate where awareness of risk is heightened, in the context of a society characterised by new notions of risk and danger (Beck, 1992). It is a society concerned with actuarial calculation of risk and its reduction and/or elimination yet one in which new risks become increasingly difficult to manage (Giddens, 1991; Parton, 1996b; Ginsburg, 1998). Much care management assessment focuses on the degree of risk in which a person is placed; indeed, this governs the 'eligibility criteria' for services. Hence risk was the aspect of the person's situation which became the focus of assessments, rather than a part of the broader picture. The eligibility criteria, which determine whether people will receive a service, label and pathologise people in order to fit them to the criteria. During the research it was observed that this labelling and pathologising was epitomised by the use of a computerised assessment form which had a mandatory section for listing risk and positioned 'risk factors' at the top of the 'pick lists' for identifying needs. In whatever way care managers approached their work, risk was a predominant factor that circumscribed it increasingly.

Such a focus detracts from, and is counter to, strategies for empowerment. The use of actuarial notions of risk imply that, rather like insuring a house or a car, a calculation can be made which will ensure that risk can be predicted. Such formulaic ways of working can all too easily rely solely on notions of professional expertise, taking little account of, where this is possible, a person's own views of their risk, and their own ideas for coping with them. This concern about risk to service users appears to be related directly to concern about another sphere of risk, mentioned by one of the staff quoted in Chapter 4, who said, '*don't get a complaint against yourself*'. This extent of concern with litigation was observed in a 'Duty and Referral' training course (Postle, 1999). Risk featured highly on the timetable. For example, the importance of recording was stressed as necessary in case of later litigation rather than for any other reason. In an exercise, staff were asked to list what they thought were the greatest risks to themselves in their work. Their most common responses were being sued, disciplinary action if you get it wrong; being exposed in the newspapers, complaints and criticism; and stress and illness. Fear of litigation clearly dominated, doubtless fuelled by the Local Authority's own fear of the resultant disruption and expenditure. We have noted in Chapters 2 and 4 that the implementation, in October 2000, of the Human Rights Act 1998 has implications for care managers' good practice in areas such as hearing the voice of the person using services, transparency in decision-making, and accurate reporting. To date, there has not been the flood of litigation resulting from this legislation that Local Authorities feared. However, as the Association of Directors of Social Services London chairperson, Anthony Douglas, has warned, this should not give grounds for complacency (Unity Sale, 2001). From recent discussions with students on social work courses it would seem that, while they acknowledge that the Human Rights Act offers channels for redress and, in turn, empowerment to service users, it has added to staff fears about the effects of litigation.

Resulting from increased fears of complaint or litigation, research indicated that some care managers were adopting procedures to 'cover themselves'. As noted in Chapter 3, care managers spent an increasing amount of time on paperwork, having less time for any depth of client contact. In this climate of risk, great emphasis was placed on recording, although all care managers spoke of the difficulty of keeping their records up to date. An example of this is Elaine's comment that she would have to put a note on Miss Allen's file to the effect that she had refused services. This was seen as a way of 'covering your back' in case of any later accident or injury sustained by the person. This lack of time to work with people where risks have been identified is likely to result, as in Miss Allen's situation, in their being left at risk. Alternatively, services may be provided in a short-termist 'quick fix-it' way which does little to enhance the person's own coping skills and, instead, is more likely to make them increasingly dependent on services.

An example of the ways in which the *minimal services and maximal dependency* described by Shakespeare at the start of this chapter (Shakespeare, 2000, p. 57) militated against empowerment is given in the following example:

Norah, visiting Mrs Lyndon-Jones, explained that, because of budgetary cutbacks, she would have to reduce the time a paid carer spent with Mrs Lyndon-Jones, taking her shopping. Norah discussed whether a volunteer could do the shopping for her instead. Mrs Lyndon-Jones was understandably disappointed by this, saying that her shopping trips were one of the few times she left her flat and, by going with a carer, she was able to choose the goods herself.

This situation was constructed as Mrs Lyndon-Jones' problem alone, rather than one that many elderly people experience. With a less individualistic approach, time to think creatively and a less market-driven environment, the situation could be resolved differently creating less dependency and with Mrs Lyndon-Jones exercising considerably more control over at least one aspect of her life.

The person's absence from decisions made about them, including decisions made about their degree of risk, is epitomised in this description of a hospital discharge planning meeting:

> *Amanda attended a discharge planning meeting at the community hospital. Mrs Atkins, 86, had been recovering from a fractured neck of femur and was due to go home. The meeting was attended by 8 hospital staff members: doctor (chair), two physiotherapists, two occupational therapists, two nurses (neither of whom was Mrs Atkins' named primary nurse) and the hospital social worker. Mrs Atkins' didn't attend the meeting, but her son did, and Amanda and Mrs Atkins' son relayed the decisions reached to her after the meeting. In talking to Amanda later, she told me that Mrs Atkins was also on a Care Programme Approach (CPA) and so had a Community Psychiatric Nurse (CPN). A CPA meeting was due but couldn't be combined with the discharge meeting, and the CPN wasn't invited to the latter.*

The diverse and fragmented nature of the human condition, and the lack of cohesion reflected in the pluralist professional responses to it, are exemplified in this description. We described the difficulties of multi-disciplinary working in Chapter 4. Nonetheless, some care managers welcomed opportunities for multi-disciplinary work, thinking that it could enhance different skills and approaches, and prevent people from being referred from one agency to another with the likelihood of duplication, overlap and confusion for clients and staff alike. In Mrs Atkins' case, however, it seemed that her differing identities as an elderly woman, a mother, a home-owner, a person with physical health problems and a person with a degree of mental frailty, were fragmented and multiplied in the meeting in which 9 professionals debated her care. The meeting failed to address her situation with any sense of cohesion, exemplified by the absence of the CPN and her named nurse. Above all, Mrs Atkins herself was absent, and only her son attended from her informal support network. Such meetings perpetuate a modernist view of professionals as the experts in the situation, dwelling on problematic issues rather than strengths, and seeking formal, organisational solutions rather than any from informal networks (Fawcett, 1998). Amanda commented that holistic approaches to care management were a *myth*, epitomising feelings expressed by several care managers that the cohesive image of care management, neatly shown as a 7 stage process (SSI and SWSG, 1991a) proved very different from the realities with which they worked.

Care managers' responses to their work: coping with its ambiguities and tensions

As described in Chapter 5, research indicated that care managers dealt with the ambiguities and tensions inherent in their work in differing ways

(Gorman, 1999b; Postle, 1999). For some there was a sense that they were trying to deconstruct their work to examine what the task might now be or how they might do it. Direct work with people remained the aspect of their work that care managers found most satisfying:

Sometimes there is job satisfaction, yes, but I think a lot of the time ... a lot of the time is stressful [The good days are made by] ... probably contact with the clients, going out and doing the visits and some ... I mean, good things happen.

However, as budgets tightened, this sense of satisfaction from direct work was tempered by an increasing frustration about checking what care would be allowed:

I still get a great deal of satisfaction from the work but the frustration is trying to fight a battle when you get back here.

These frustrations contributed to care managers feeling demoralised. As the following comment from a care manager indicates, their confidence became eroded and this made it hard to remain optimistic, especially when such feelings were widely held:

That's the crux, really – just very low morale. I mean, to be honest, I find it doesn't bear ... I can't ... I don't want to think too much about what might happen in the hope that it mightn't. As I said, the pendulum might swing back. I just have to take it almost day to day and see how it comes. But the team – it is poor morale and that slowly starts to erode your ... confidence. It's very hard to keep plodding away and keep cheerful about things if you can see your colleagues sinking.

For some care managers, as we saw in Chapter 4, their only way of coping with the work was to behave in a way that could be viewed as subversive. They did this by doing what one care manager described as:

undercover work, [done] behind the system's back, if you like. Trying to do some social work in my spare time but I'll have to nip back and get on and do the work on the computer or whatever.

This *undercover* work comprised the kind of client contact exemplified by the quotations from care managers in Chapter 4.

While many care managers were trying to understand the changed nature of their work, for some this was a process they did not see as relevant, or possibly felt they had undertaken as far as they could. Instead of questioning what they're doing, as one of their team managers said, they appeared simply to be getting on with the job. One of the staff, working as a 'duty officer' at the first point of contact people had with the Social Services office, had found a way of coping with her work that no longer involved questioning its inherent dissonance. It is epitomised in her comments:

I just think I'm a DSS officer and I'm a bureaucrat ... probably a bit more compassionate ... [Duty is] front line and my aim is to get rid of as many referrals as possible ... try to divert them somewhere else before I even have to deal with them ... Get rid of it, that's my aim.

In Chapter 4 we described some of the mechanisms that 'street level bureaucrats' employ in order to help them cope with complex tasks and limited resources. Lipsky includes among these *husbanding resources* and the development of a *client-processing mentality* (Lipsky, 1980). The dilemma he describes 'street level bureaucrats' as facing applied to the way some care managers saw their work:

The existential problem for street level bureaucrats is that with any single client they probably could interact flexibly and responsively. But if they did this with too many clients their capacity to respond flexibly would disappear. One might think of each client as, in a sense, seeking to be the one for whom an exception is made, a favor [sic] done, an indiscretion overlooked, a regulation ignored. (Lipsky, 1980, p 99)

The level of routinisation that can result from trying to cope with high workloads and reduced resources was exemplified by a member of staff on a training course, who commented:

Some people in our office are saying, "If we haven't got it [referring to money], they can't bloody have it".

The person quoting this expressed concern, saying that she found such sentiments worrying because of their apparent distancing from people and their difficulties.

In contrast to the duty social worker, the care manager quoted here was happy with the job, finding it satisfying to be able to help people:

I find it quite satisfying ... in this area, we're getting our resources needs led and that's making it a bit easier. I find that, with most of my clients, I'm able to give them what they want ... I haven't had to really turn anybody down so that's quite satisfying really ... I just love it. I love the job. I always have done so ... I like people. I like meeting new people and of course I do the sight loss courses for people who are partially sighted and that's a satisfying course – that's just brilliant. People gain so much from it that you feel so good.

While most care managers identified positive aspects of the job, such as better services and enabling very dependent elderly people to remain in their homes, this was usually tinged with disappointment and frustration about other aspects of the work. Few staff spoke with similar enthusiasm, and this person's enthusiasm appears to stem from an uncomplicated view of caring which can identify it uncritically as an unquestionably 'good thing' (Fox, 1995, p. 115), without seeing its complexities and contradictions. Most staff, as we noted in Chapter 3, described more of their time being taken up with the bureaucratic tasks that increasingly shaped and determined the care management process. Such processes lead to the construction of people's situations in ways that define them as problematic in order that, in turn, their needs can be defined within given criteria. These approaches not only disempower service users; they also limit workers' scope and creativity in ways that they too experience as disempowering.

Implications of demoralised workers doing demoralising work in times of uncertainty and ambiguity
When we set care management in its societal context we can discover some explanation for the ambiguity and uncertainty characterising the work. 'Modern' society could be described as characterised by post-Enlightenment notions of certainty, progress and trust in the validity of scientific discovery. In contrast, the twentieth-century was marked by an increased questioning of whether rationality/reason can lead to truth/knowledge. Two world wars, the Holocaust, the bombing of Hiroshima and Nagasaki, and the lasting threat of nuclear annihilation, among other events and threats, have called into question the optimism generated by the Enlightenment. They have highlighted the oppressive nature of its rationality and the limitations of its ambitions and promises (Harvey, 1989, Smart, 1993). 'Postmodern' society can be seen as facing up to the consequences of modernity and hence characterised by greater uncertainty, ambivalence, ambiguity and contingency. Features of contemporary society include its ephemeral and fragmented nature, the compression of space and time (as in the operation of international money markets), the distrust of grand theories – such as Christianity or Marxism – as being capable of offering global explanations, and a sense of disembeddedness in which contexts shift and change (Harvey, 1989; Smart, 1993; Appignanesi *et al.*, 1995).

Universalising notions/grand theory can no longer be relied on to provide explanations or as a basis for constructing policy or theory, and the validity of any all-embracing, universal theory is questioned increasingly. Currently the picture becomes more one of pastiche, collage, plurality and fragmentation characterised by variety, contingency, relativism and ambivalence (Harvey, 1989; Bauman, 1992; Howe, 1994). 'Citizenship' has taken on an individualised meaning in an increasingly decentralised and localised society (Lash and Urry, 1994). As we noted above when considering whether care management is 'empowering older people or exacerbating dependency', with increasing uncertainty there is greater emphasis on risk (Giddens, 1991; Beck, 1992).

It can be argued that social work was born, and continues to exist, in the space between public and private, where it both occupies and attempts to mediate between state and civil, excluded and mainstream, respectable and deviant/dangerous, wealth and poverty, those with rights and those without, those within and those outside the market economy, the autonomous/free and the governed (Clarke, 1993; Parton, 1994; Cree, 1995; Jordan, 1997). This offers some explanation of the position of tension care managers experience as they attempt to mediate between these dichotomous positions and find themselves struggling with ambiguities, such as resolving the outcomes of constrained resources, with a wish to provide a service, or undertaking bureaucratic tasks with less time to engage in therapeutic encounters with people. This position of ambiguity is also one of indirect social regulation, in which the care manager maintains a social policing role in, for example, the assessment of risk with elderly, confused people.

Lack of certainty has not resulted in an end to a search for truth in the field of care management but rather a plurality of searches such as different forms of working and a plethora of systems, guidance and procedures which are constantly subject to revision and change. These procedures can also be seen as a means of governing/regulating the profession. Current practice is characterised by increasingly greater degrees of uncertainty, contingency and ambiguity. Fragmentation is characterised in care management's lack of a unifying theoretical base and its diffusion of theory.

There would appear to be clear links between a workforce perceiving itself to be deskilled and demoralised, operating a reductionist process of assessment in a climate in which managerialist and financial concerns dominate, and the quality of service that older people receive. Focusing largely on crisis elements of the work appeared to be demoralising for staff, many of whom could see the effects of what they considered to be very short-termist policy. Their lowered morale must, in turn, affect how they work with people. For example Rosemary, whose work with Mrs Lindford was described above as an example – albeit in a small way – of empowerment, resigned as a care manager, and commented in an interview shortly before she left:

> *I suppose that's* [referring to contact with clients] *why you go into social work and that's where the satisfaction comes from ... that's diminished, for me, there's very little satisfaction. There are bits, but it comes from when I'm doing social work. This other stuff isn't social work is it? It's care management, which I think is just a different job.*

Her comments are reminiscent of what Blaug, quoted in Chapter 3, was writing about when he said that instrumentalist procedures helped bad social workers and hindered good ones.

Care managers considered that their autonomy was being eroded, which led to most of them feeling a degree of de-skilling and devaluing where they formerly felt trusted and valued, and some even questioned whether it was worth continuing in the work. Overtly this reduction in autonomy appeared to be caused by reduced budgets and to a desire for financial accountability, but it also implied greater regulation of care managers. Such regulation is a hallmark of managerialism, positioning team managers in the roles of gate-keeper and decision-maker, and removing them yet further from expertise in the day-to-day work of the frontline staff. This was how one team manager described this:

People feel their autonomy is undermined ... that's been one of the things they like about the job, that you're a professional, you've got autonomy, you make your decision. Now it's restricted. They can't get in, assess the needs and say, 'This is what this person's got to have ...' and go ahead with it ... If you can't do that, you've got to say, 'Oh well ... I'm sorry. We've got to wait ... go to panel' ... If you take that autonomy away ... you feel you're being devalued and not used properly so I think that's a very serious thing ... we do all feel de-skilled by that ... controlled.

Some care managers expressed concerns that, while their clients might not notice any deterioration in service, their own needs as professional staff were not being met. It would seem, however, that as Simiç, quoting Smith *et al.*, has shown (Smith *et al.*, 1995; Simiç, 1997): 'Service users missed just those elements of social work, the interpersonal and empathic, that were being written out of professional practice by process-oriented and mechanistic care management' (Simiç, 1997, p. 2). Indications from a recent Social Services Inspectorate (SSI) report further indicate this concentration on processes and service responses, rather than skilful, analytical assessment that would benefit clients. The report's authors write:

Casework as part of care management or direct work is often not present even when the situation requires it – for example – services are often the only (although necessary) response to a person coming to terms with being at home after discharge from hospital. (DOH/SSI, 1999, para 1.24)

The inevitable conclusions are that social work's traditional position of tension and ambiguity has been emphasised by recent changes (Postle, 2002). The problems caused by the degree of change have been compounded by the way in which all levels of management have managed it, resulting in disempowerment, rather than empowerment, of staff (Smale and Tuson, 1992). It becomes clear that, if staff perceive themselves as being disempowered, they are not likely to be able to lift their heads sufficiently to consider strategies, such as those we have referenced in the box below, to empower the people with whom they work. These strategies may seem a small start and run the risk of tokenism, but nonetheless they could form the start of a shift in thinking and operation away from managerialist, procedurally-driven, defensive practice. Hence we list them here:

Checklist for empowerment strategies

- Learn from people using services what empowerment means for them rather than imposing understandings which may be meaningless or wrong.

- Work with the reality of empowerment, not the rhetoric.

- Be alert to ways of working that exacerbate people's dependency and militate against empowerment.

- Demoralised and disempowered staff are unlikely to be able to empower others.

- For guidance on providing good practice and responsive services, see:

    - Morris, J (1995) *The Power to Change*, London, Kings Fund Centre. pp. 39–40

    - Bornat, J. (1997a) 'Anthology: Charters' in *Community Care: a Reader* (eds) Bornat, J, Johnson, J, Pereira, C, Pilgrim, D and Williams, F) London, Macmillan, pp 266–76

Suggestions for further reading about empowerment

Braye, S and Preston-Shoot, M (1995) *Empowering Practice in Social Care* Buckingham, Open University Press

Burke, B and Harrison, P (1998) 'Anti-oppressive practice' in (eds, Adams, R, Dominelli, L and Payne, M, *Social Work: Themes, Issues and Critical Debates* London, Macmillan

Croft, S and Beresford, P (2000) 'Empowerment' in (ed) Davies, M, *Blackwell Encyclopaedia of Social Work* Oxford, Blackwell

Morris, J (1991) *Pride Against Prejudice* London, The Women's Press

Oliver, M (1996) *Understanding Disablitiy: from theory to practice* London, Macmillan

Servian, R (1996) *Theorising Empowerment: individual power and community care* Bristol, Policy Press

Shakespeare, T (2000) *Help* Birmingham, Venture Press

Smale, G, Tuson, G, with Biehal, N and Marsh, P (1993) *Empowerment, Assessment, Care Management and the Skilled Worker* London, HMSO

Chapter 6
Conclusion

An overview

The vision of community care has, in many respects, been distorted into the reality of care management. The community care revolution of the late 1980s and early 1990s, which was conceived from the political conviction that the welfare state was too costly to run and the answer lay in market enterprise, had a huge impact on how individuals experience welfare services at the start of the twenty-first century. At the same time, it is possible to acknowledge that community care has always been in a state of change. Certainly de-institution-alisation was not a new phenomenon. One difference lies in the nature and pace of the change that was experienced throughout the welfare system. Our view is that the changes that have led to the transformation of community care into care management represent a distortion of the original vision, and this distor-tion can be viewed in both negative and positive terms. This concluding chapter aims to explain some of those problems and possibilities.

We argue that the reality of community care – that is how this concept is currently experienced by users, carers, workers and organisations – has for the most part been operationalised within a configuration called care management. Care management became the vehicle in which the realities of community care policies were spelt out and, as will become apparent in this concluding chapter, these influences remain dominant in the current drive towards primary care in the community. Since the research for this book was undertaken, the policy agenda has shifted even further towards joint working between health and social services. Decision-making about the use of resources has become localised around Primary Care Groups and Trusts, with the prospect of Care Trusts encompassing both health and welfare responsibilities.

In this book we have identified differences between the reality and rhetoric of community care as experienced through the system of care man-agement. Sadly, we have evidenced a picture of service-driven assessment carried out by a largely demoralised work force. The context has been rationing, and managerial control and audit. Central to this process has been the care manager, who is usually a social worker.

Care managers as employees within welfare agencies have been, and continue to be, aware of the application of market principles to their work. Through contact with these mechanisms, care managers' roles have formed part of a wider change process. Since the implementation of care management in

1993, a reconfiguration has taken place in the way that social workers working in care management view their work and their professional identity. The application of social construction theory (Berger and Luckman, 1966) is helpful in recognising that, as role performers, the conduct of care managers in a welfare bureaucracy becomes susceptible to enforcement. Compliance or non-compliance with socially-defined role standards ceases to be optional and there is a threat of sanction for non-compliance. At times, care managers appear to be skating on thin ice; there is an awareness of legal threats and sanctions if 'mistakes' are made, and this can lead to defensive practice. What the care manager learns as part of this process is significant, because:

> *By virtue of the roles he* [sic] *plays the individual is inducted into specific areas of socially objectivated knowledge, not only in the narrower cognitive sense, but also in the sense of the 'knowledge' of norms, values and even emotions.* (Berger and Luckman, 1966, p. 94)

As discussed in Chapter 3, the emotional labour of the care manager in the context of the commodification of welfare (Gorman, 2000b) is part of the reality that both users of welfare and care managers have experienced. It is acknowledged that the views of care managers themselves are only one part of a bigger story, because within a social constructivist framework there is both similarity and difference. Human reality as a socially-constructed reality relates to understandings of knowledge, and it is the way that such knowledge is harnessed and developed in context that is the essential debate. Parallels can be made for users of services because, as we discussed in Chapter 5, the language of empowerment has not been a lived experience for many recipients of welfare, not least because its language has generally been inaccessible to them.

The influence of the market on welfare and the new public-sector management that developed in the 1990s had an impact on the identity and role of the care manager both in terms of tasks and in the way that the labour process developed, influencing care managers' agendas in terms of priorities, and consequently their relationships with service users. The care managers' narratives in the research that forms the basis of this book bears a strong similarity to that of Lipsky's (1980) *Street Level Bureaucrats* in the way that the tensions generated by decision-making processes affected power dynamics between the users of services and the care managers, with the potential for disempowerment all round. As we discussed in Chapters 3 and 4, there was evidence of inherent conflicts passed down to the practice level for resolution or irresolution, with care managers modifying their roles and their objectives to reduce gaps between available resources and achieving objectives. Resistance to these forces were apparent, with some significant discourses emerging about loss of autonomy and the need to be accountable. Accountability was defined less in terms of professional accountability than as the monitoring and audit of activity in which episodes of time or unit costs were the predominant norm. Such experiences have in some instances enhanced the tenacity of some workers. Take the view of one experienced practitioner, for example:

> *Senior practitioners in the game for a long time have felt under siege for the past few years. They are beginning to emerge and say 'Look, hang on, this is still social work, there is nothing different in this'. I am getting the feeling that social workers are proud of their background, they are proud of what they are doing, proud of the social work skills that they have, and that they are relieved to know that they can still use those skills.*

The situation of professional practice (Schön, 1987; Schön, 1992) emerges as one characterised by complexity, instability, uncertainty, uniqueness and value conflict, and one in which the stakes can be high for the service user in terms of the quality of life they might experience as a result of the decisions of the care manager. As discussed in Chapter 4, such decisions, often taken in a climate of risk, are made by personnel who, from their accounts of their activities and perception of role, can make a legitimate claim to expertise. Some evidence from care managers, in this book and elsewhere, suggests a resistance to attempts to fragment the care manager role, and a picture emerges of work in which continuity and some strategic vision are important factors. For example, the case studies reported by Goss and Miller indicate clear possibilities for user involvement and empowerment. They demonstrate examples of care management work moving from a standpoint of 'them and us' to 'us and us', which gave credibility to the least considered care manager role, that of service users acting as their own care managers (Goss and Miller, 1995). Nonetheless, as we noted in Chapter 5, Hugman (1994) has warned that the managerial concerns inherent in the community care reforms could reinforce and perpetuate ageism by routinising the work with older people and doing nothing to address the status of social work practice with them.

One deeply-etched picture that emerges is of care managers as welfare bureaucrats with a role that increasingly is being circumscribed by the policy drive to pin down work activity into units that can be audited. However, rather than being unidimensional, the picture is a hologram, with another perspective being the care manager as expert engaging with users in a climate of uncertainty and risk, drawing on professional skills with the aim of meeting users' needs within the boundaries of available resources. The reinforcement of either perspective in practice depends on individual perception, attitude and strategy intent. The development of care management, a legitimate activity in public welfare, has had a significant impact on the professional identity of social workers working with adults in community care.

Yet we have evidence of a number of positive aspects in community care in transition. In summary, they involve:

- more acceptance of the user as being central to the care compact;
- potential for innovation in service provision; and
- the opportunity to develop strong community networks.

The growth of the market in welfare offers opportunities for innovative practice if there is a genuine choice and facilities are available. As discussed in Chapters 4 and 5, it is possible to create autonomy by harnessing potentially enabling strategies such as direct payments. The contradictions in the notion of empowerment expressed as social exclusion, polarisation and marginalisation do not have to be reinforced by the process of care management. The issue remains, however, about how best to facilitate empowerment in an inherently contradictory system where the state inevitably controls the purse strings – this is perhaps the ultimate 'Catch 22'. Moving towards that goal rather than expecting to achieve it within a given timescale may be the appropriate mindset to adopt. The care manager as an enabler is a realistic phenomenon as long as the processes are transparent and the goals are shared. However, it is unrealistic to deny the power of welfare organisations as arms of the state bureaucracy, and in turn the power of those who act as agents.

The complexity of interventions and their range and number, together with the perspectives of those involved have, in terms of their inherent uncertainty, characterised welfare work. This has happened specifically with care management as the visible expression of community care. At the same time, the power cultures in welfare bureaucracies have been hierarchical and rule-bound with characteristics of problem avoidance, individualism, low avoidance of uncertainty and, as has been discussed previously, has been subjected to a 'new managerialism' that favoured short-term planning and 'macho' management styles. The dilemma created by the divergence of these approaches can generate persistent problems over meeting the needs of users of the services.

Collaboration in community care needs to be explored for its potential for empowerment (Gorman *et al.*, 1996). One interpretation is for social services and health agencies to work together to deliver better services to users in their own homes. The intention of policy-makers is that agencies should enter into collaborative arrangements, and thus by pooling resources, skills and ideas, agencies would have the potential to create new and better services. To work in collaboration with service users means being aware of the values, knowledge and skills that people possess by enabling them to achieve their own goals (Trevillion, 1993). Both the personal and organisational dynamics of working together reflect the power dimensions that are part of the process of collaboration.

> *Collaboration and conflict often exist side by side – they are part of a process. Collaboration is a realistic term to apply to the changing context of health and social care when it is conceived as a term that denotes the process of working towards achieving shared goals rather than being seen solely as a functional outcome. Collaboration is an emergent process; it relates to a multi-dimensional, cyclical and iterative development that forms part of the contemporary reality of practice in community care and primary care.* (Gorman, 2000a, p. 69)

Quality outcomes for service users means that those involved in the assessment, planning and delivery of community care services need to work together. This process is difficult when a workforce is demoralised. The empirical evidence that forms the basis of this book points to a crisis in the professional identity of social workers who operationalise care management. The next part of the conclusion discusses how factors relating to community care in transition trigger a consideration of the need for deconstruction and reconstruction of the nature of social work.

Implications for the future: deconstructing and reconstructing social work
When describing social work the care managers interviewed usually spoke as if this was a discrete entity that had been lost in the transition to care management (Gorman, 1999b; Postle, 1999). This, together with their dichotomous oppositional positioning of social work against care management, is understandable given the radical changes they had experienced in their work and its location at a transitional phase from modern to postmodern. It would be easy to dismiss their comments as nostalgia, but an alternative explanation could be that staff were using what Giddens describes as the internally referential development of the self: 'The creation of a personal belief system by means of which the individual acknowledges that "his first loyalty is to himself". The key reference points are "set from the inside" in terms of how the individual constructs/reconstructs his life history' (Giddens, 1991, p. 80).

Hence staff constructed their identities reflexively as care managers and, when their work became increasingly at odds with this construction, they organised memories of their work congruently with their expectations of what it should have been.

The diverse and contested nature of social work was not the focus of the interviews; rather, the emphasis was on the contrast with care management. In making this contrast, care managers talked about the elements of social work that they thought had been reduced or lost in the transition. Hence they described the loss of therapeutic elements such as counselling, listening and support, which were also aspects of their work that they found to be rewarding and satisfying. These elements were collapsed under the heading 'social work' as if they constituted that role in an uncontested and non-problematic way.

Taking such a definition of social work as a given fails to problematise and deconstruct its nature, thereby not yielding it to critical examination. In failing to do this, the diverse elements of social work have not been scrutinised in the context of its societal location. Lacking this critical examination, social work, in the move to care management, has taken on attributes of contemporary society, apparently uncritically. Hence care management has evolved as a highly individualistic response to problem solving, creating individual packages of care for individual people within a managerialist and market-driven ethos. The possibility of working in less individualistic ways would necessitate operating in a manner that challenges this prevailing ethos. The threat to the continuation of social work with adults is that it continues to fail to challenge this ethos and becomes subsumed by managerialist and market-driven agendas.

Like social work, care management is in a process of being, rather than an entity that has become. As such, as well as the threat outlined above, there are seeds of opportunity for further challenge and change, and for the possibility of a reinvention/reconceptualisation/reconstruction of social work/care management, representing the new theories that Kuhn describes as generally preceded by a period of pronounced professional uncertainty (Kuhn, 1962, p. 67). This would involve the users and practitioners of care management jointly and confidently defining its role in contemporary society rather than this being defined by the prevailing ethos. Such a reconstruction would prove empowering for both users of services and staff.

Within social work, and within care management, there are diverse elements, with underlying theoretical assumptions, all of which can be deconstructed and then reconstructed and assessed for their potential in addressing the social problems of service users. This goes beyond taking a prescriptive stance of 'what works', which lends itself all too readily to a positivist and questionable interpretation of evidence-based practice (for example, Sheldon, 1986). Rather, it involves deconstructing social work to ascertain content, meanings, scope and nature. This includes an examination of the constituents of social work, its theories, values, knowledge, skills and practices and, as Pease and Fook suggest, their underlying premises in ways that acknowledge and incorporate tensions between different, even opposing, strands (Pease and Fook, 1999). It would involve examining where social work practice was flawed – such as in its tendency to a paternalistic nature or its failure to make alliances, both with people who use its services and with other bodies who work with them – as well as its strengths. The diverse and eclectic nature of social work practice, encompassing the therapeutic and emotional as well as the radical and political, its ability to work with the individual as well as with the wider networks and communities and its potential for drawing upon a broad and diverse knowledge base need to be deconstructed and valued equally rather than seen as vying for position as the best, or only, form of practice.

While social work has tended to be apologetic for, and defensive of, its eclectic nature, by deconstructing this eclecticism and then reconstructing those elements of social work which can be used to meet peoples' differing needs effectively and appropriately, care management could become assertive about its body of values, knowledge and skills. There are implications for educating care managers if they are not to feel ill-equipped to undertake the tasks ahead when they qualify. While there is clearly no role for university departments to be involved in teaching students how to complete forms and manage information technology (IT) programmes, curriculum development should ensure that staff are as well equipped as possible to deal with the ambiguities and tensions with which the work inevitably presents them. Any developments which use a 'both/and' rather than an 'either/or' approach to maintaining academic standards while meeting employers' needs must be beneficial (Postle, 2001).

From our research, it became apparent that most care managers had a sense that something was wrong with current practice but, while they were able to describe this, and to compare it with former practice, they did not articulate it theoretically (Postle, 1999). In a climate in which outcomes of community care policies tend to be defined as those that are easily measurable, success can be inferred from the increasing number of people with high levels of personal assistance needs who are now being maintained in the community. Such outcome measures ignore the views of those people with lower needs, and users' opinions about the quality of service received (Nocon and Qureshi, 1996). Hence care managers, lacking the theoretical understanding with which to critique such policies or their operationalisation, appear to be levelling unfocused criticisms at a system that is working. As we have demonstrated in this book, a fuller theoretical understanding of the societal condition in which care management is operating, and of how societal characteristics are reflected in care management practice, would equip care managers to evaluate and critique their practice and the operation of the agencies within which they work with greater confidence.

Implications for practice, in addition to those outlined above, include questioning the current location of social work primarily within Local Authorities. While social work/care management will inevitably be subject to budgetary constraints wherever it is located, its location within Local Authorities driven largely by a managerialist and market ethos (Syrett *et al.*, 1997) appears to be detrimental to its continuing professional identity. Consideration of the advantages and disadvantages of other practice locations, such as within primary health care teams, may offer scope for the continuation of a discrete professional identity and practice as well as the ability to work with people with varying levels of need, rather than being constrained by the rigidity of eligibility criteria (Lymbery, 1999; Simiç, 1997). Practice approaches that encompass a broader, community perspective, rather than concentrating solely on individualised work, may offer more imaginative ways of meeting users' and carers' needs (Smale *et al.*, 2000).

The findings in the research that generated this book, and the conclusions of the national surveys of care management (DOH and Challis, 1994; DOH/SSI, 1998), indicate that complex care management requires professional skills. The 1998 Study of Care Management Arrangements commissioned by the DOH concluded:

The visits showed that there is scope for authorities to adopt a more differentiated set of arrangements in order to more effectively manage volume and to make efficient use of skills available. Thus different processes and different skill mixes can be adopted for different stages and different levels of complexity. (DOH/SSI, 1998, 3.12)

The acknowledgement of different levels of complexity in care management work and the need for care managers to have skills to enable them to cope with complexity leads us to consider the nature of the skills required. There are specific skills a care manager requires, such as professional assessment skills, the ability to negotiate and work collaboratively with others, and to manage conflict when it arises (Gorman, 2000b). Care managers need to be able to plan their work, and plan and manage the organisation of care episodes in a context of change and scarce resources.

Community care in transition – towards learning organisations in health and social care?

It has become accepted increasingly within the public sector that the training and development of staff is linked in some way to organisational effectiveness, and that priorities for training needs must be related to organisational goals. The establishment of the Training Organisation for the Personal Social Services (TOPSS), recognised initially for the period 1998–2001, has a remit to oversee the strategic planning of education, training and qualification for the sector.

Various concepts predominate in the aims of TOPSS, including the development of a more *competent* workforce. The notion of competence can be interpreted in a number of ways. In the context of community care, a narrow interpretation that limits the term to the achievement of competencies leads to a reductionist approach that could stifle innovation (Gorman, 2000b). Problems to be tackled are acknowledged as a workforce that is sometimes ill-prepared for the complex problems they face, a fragmented relationship between policy development and the workforce skills to implement; and an often poor understanding of workforce management issues. This initiative has run parallel with Social Services performance frameworks (DOH, 1999). Local authorities are expected to compare their performance with other authorities through 'performance' and 'best value' indicators, with performance reviews being undertaken within a five-year cycle, to encourage continuous improvement. While acknowledging that agencies may need to do better than at present, another phase of monitoring of performance is unlikely to be welcomed by the front-line staff, such as care managers. The continuing trends towards auditing and performance review within health and social services organisations, intensified by the Labour Government in power at the time of writing, appear to be juxtaposed with a continuing recognition for 'professional' social work in *Modernising Social Services* (DOH, 1998b), albeit this appears to be in a more regulated format, with an endorsement for the continuation of the role of the care manager in complex care management (DOH, 1998d).

As the authors of this book concluded from their empirical research, moves towards improving standards in practice are linked to the education and training of the workforce. Evaluation of such training, it is argued, should be concerned not only with the skills, knowledge and attitudes an individual acquires through the learning process, but also with changes in work performance; although such a leap is often difficult to determine with any certainty in the short term, if at all. The paradigm of measurement and the implication of certainty about learning pervades the literature on training in social and health services, for example: 'Training should increase the effectiveness of individual workers, so evaluating training depends on setting clear criteria against which the changes in effectiveness can be measured' (Bramley and Pahl, 1996, p. 37). There is a general acknowledgement that the contexts in which people work are relevant to developing them as a workforce. The concept of the learning organisation, while it does not appear to have been linked explicitly to care management as an activity, is important in that it focuses the agenda on quality outcomes.

A move away from individual competencies to core organisational competencies reflects a notion of 'communities of practice' but is likely to be configured within a regime of audit and monitoring (Power, 1997). A relatively small proportion of the workforce may need crucial skills for a particular area of work and therefore a blanket re-skilling of employees is likely to be inappropriate and inefficient. Nonetheless, this approach is being attempted. One of the problems of a general approach that aims to up-skill the workforce is that individuals' willingness to engage and invest in training is limited if they cannot see personal gain from the training and do not know whether the employer recognises the value of such training.

The requirement for social work managers to recognise the need for staff training is a significant issue for the social services workforce (Balloch *et al.*, 1995; Balloch *et al.*, 1997) and in the mid-1990s appeared to be weak in relation to the discrete area of collaborative work in community care; managers in both health and social services did not see the need as a priority (Gorman, 1994). The Labour Government's policy intentions for greater flexibility of working between health and social services do, however, imply a greater imperative for employers to get involved in lifelong learning and joint education initiatives (DOH, 1998b) and these aspects of current policy.

The notion that there can be 'learning organisations' is one that has gathered momentum with the development of an understanding of the term 'lifelong learning', which reinforces a social-market model of education and training. As Hyland (1994) comments, 'lifelong learning' and 'the learning organisation' are problem terms in that they can become powerfully persuasive slogans that mask critical differences between approaches to learning ranging from economic utility models to ones that favour critical practice and incorporate social change. The learning processes in a learning organisation are problem-orientated, and in this respect they differ from a prescriptive organisation (such as within a bureaucracy), which is designed to prevent the occurrence of problems: 'In a learning organisation problems are seen as interesting indicators of changes that might be needed' (Swieringa and Wierdsma, 1992, p. 73).

Within such a model, learning takes place on the job, and the processes are linked to work. The focus of a 'learning organisation' is directed towards developing staff in 'learning to learn', called meta-learning. This approach may be suited to small companies, but may be less appropriate for a bureaucracy such as Social Services, the transformation of which would be more complicated than a modification of its organisational principles. However, approaches to lifelong learning within organisations can reflect the requirements of particular professional and regulatory bodies such as the Nursing and Midwifery Council (NMC) and General Social Care Council (GSCC). In the conclusions to their research into graduate employment, Harvey *et al.*, (1997) state that continuous learning is something cited repeatedly by employers and recent graduates as an essential and integral part of working, highlighting the need to constantly develop in order to keep up with the demands of the job.

Learning for complex care management is an activity that requires the application of values in practice, which by its very nature cannot wholly be an individualised activity. As has already been discussed in this book, it demands problematisation and decision-making in risk situations and in a climate of uncertainty. It is an activity that requires knowledge and skills in context. Fisher (1997) discusses the kind of knowledge required for social work practice in community care, but not specifically care management, and he draws a distinction between evidence-based and knowledge-based practice and between knowledge for understanding and that designed to underpin intervention. Fisher (1997) considers that educators must review and adapt an existing skill base to develop participative techniques. Also that the core of the approach is a value base and only when this is adopted as a set of principles does it matter how to make it work in practice. He highlights that the key knowledge base for community care derives from negotiation and gives the example of the assessment process (part of care management). In the context of care management it is interesting to note that in the research of Lewis *et al.*, (1995) they concluded that one reason why care-purchasing decisions were pushed up the decision-making ladder was a lack of negotiating skills among care managers. Other key skill areas for complex care management include collaboration, negotiation, conflict management, evaluation and critical reflection (Gorman, 1999b, 2000b).

Fisher (1997) believes that a knowledge base for social work in community care that includes such general principles as empowerment needs constantly to be re-examined and reinvented in the light of the experiences of the people whose welfare it is intended to enhance. In his paper, Fisher concludes that:

Social work in community care is an intellectually demanding practical activity where knowledge is adapted flexibly and rapidly to underpin intervention and where broad principles are adapted to specific circumstances. This is a very different vision of social work knowledge for community care than currently characterises UK debate. It contrasts with the competency-based approach to the knowledge base which has tended to lead to reductionist lists of abilities to be added into the educational programme

(Fisher, 1997, p. 26).

For Eraut (1994), the term 'continuing professional development' is preferable to 'continuing professional education' because, in his view, such a term incorporates learning that may take place in courses, for example in a university, with learning that takes place in the workplace. A problem common to professional and post-qualification education is how to ensure that learning is relevant to work, and consequently in this context that the quality of welfare work enhances the lives of citizens. An educational process needs to be developed that is not dictated solely by employer-led outcomes but considers the personal development needs of employees as people who wish to contribute to the welfare project through their work capacity. As skill requirements shift and knowledge needs become more volatile, education and training has to try to keep abreast of such changes. Continuous professional development involves the systematic maintenance, improvement and broadening of knowledge and skill, and the development of personal qualities to carry out the work role (Walsh and Woodward, 1989). Current policy and practice initiatives related to the future of qualifying and post-qualifying social work training (CCETSW, 1998), training for care management (DOH/SSI, 1997; DOH/SSI, 1998) and current monitoring processes such as the RAP's project 1998/9 (referrals, assessment and packages of care project) (DOH, 2001) are pertinent to that debate.

Learning for a work context that involves complexity, diversity and uncertainty necessitates the development and use of appropriate learning strategies and methodologies that can incorporate such notions. A model of continuing education for welfare professionals such as care managers should take into account the process of developing knowledge, understanding and skills in relation to a 'principle-centred paradigm' (Covey, 1993) — within a social context that is subject to change. Developing tools and techniques for the application of appropriate models requires evaluation over a period of time. Such techniques may include the use of learning logs or diaries, learning partners and self-assessment schedules (Gorman, 1995; Boud and Knights, 1996; Gorman, 1996a) and personal development as an explicit element of the learning process as a buffer between the worlds of work and academia. The transfer of learning from the relative safety of academia to the world of practice is tricky, as is any transfer of learning from one situation to another, even within the same context. This endorses Eraut's (1994) view that an essential element in a process of continuing personal development is learning to learn.

Bureaucracies such as Social Services Departments may be slower to adapt to such a changing environment, but nevertheless strategies that incorporate synergy, partnership and innovation to meet the service requirements of users in a climate of rationed resources need to be supported by expert practitioners who can cope with the dynamics of uncertainty, diversity and change.

Any bottom-line search for quality in care management would include consideration of the work of the care manager and the 'training' required for the job. A question that needs to be asked is what sort of 'quality' and what sort of 'training'. Quality policies take time to be put into effect in most organisations. Stages can be identified that move the organisation from minimum to ideal standards in a process of continual development (Gaster, 1995). However, such an approach demands a clarity about the nature of the quality that is being sought. A preferred vision of the future is one that acknowledges competing priorities and considers the importance of establishing a value base. Part of any drive towards improved quality is the continuing education of employees.

The empirical research into skills for care management activity endorses the view that continuing education is as much about the personal as it is about the professional (Gorman, 1999a). Just as quality itself is about negotiation between key interests, we argue that skills development for the complexities of care management requires an acknowledgement of 'higher-order' skills relating to the role of the expert in context. Personal development and growth is part of a learning process that is subtle, iterative and occasionally painful. All the more reason why employing agencies need to nurture their already-competent staff by allowing them to be experts within the boundaries of their role rather than condemning them for not conforming with often poorly-considered applications of policy directives.

Learning methodologies that are holistic and ongoing rather than reductionist, fragmented and finite need to be recognised as worthwhile by both the policy-makers and the managers who implement total quality management and the training and educational initiatives within that paradigm. This may require a significant culture shift within organisations that employ care managers, both now and in the future. A recognition that attaining quality is a collective enterprise and one that can be stultified by standardisation is part of that process.

Continuing professional development is a concept that has a resonance for health and welfare occupations. Shifting professional identities and the potential impact of the rights and responsibilities of citizens in mapping out their own futures is part of a contemporary and changing landscape that demands interdisciplinary work and collaborative effort by staff at all levels. Continuing professional development requires linkages to be established and sustained between educationists, practitioners and managers. Such connections, while they may be espoused, need to be made real and effective at both qualifying and post-qualifying levels of training and beyond.

To quote Robert Pirsig, in *Zen and the Art of Motorcycle Maintenance*:

> *The real cycle that you are working on is a cycle called yourself. The machine that appears to be "out there" and the person that appears to be "in here" are not two separate things. They grow towards Quality or fall away from Quality together* (Pirsig, 1974, p. 328).

Such a statement applies both to the continuing education of care managers and to the process and outcomes for users of the services. Community care has been transformed into care management and is likely to remain as such for some time to come. Recognising the unique views, contributions and choices of service users within the confines of the welfare system remains the major challenge. The notion of community participation needs to be embedded in enlightened and effective strategies for the continuing professional development of staff involved.

Bibliography

Appignanesi, R, Garratt, C, Sardar, Z and Curry, P (1995) *Postmodernism for Beginners* Cambridge, Icon Books

Audit Commission (1986) *Making a Reality of Community Care* London, HMSO,

Bailey, R and Brake, R (1975) *Radical Social Work* London, Edward Arnold

Baldock, J and Ungerson, C (1994) *Becoming Consumers of Community Care Householders within the Mixed Economy of Welfare* York, Joseph Rowntree Foundation

Balloch, S, Andrew, T, Ginn, G, McLean, J, Pahl, J and Williams, J (1995) *Working in the Social Services Research Summary 1* London, NISW

Balloch, S, Andrew, T, Davey, B, Dolan, L, Fisher, M, Ginn, J, McLean, J and Pahl, J (1997) *The Social Services Workforce in Transition, Research Summary 1* London, NISW

Barclay, P (1982) *Social Workers Their Roles and Tasks (The Barclay Report)* London, NISW

Barnes, M and Wistow, G (1995) *User-Orientated Community Care: an overview of findings from an evaluation of the Birmingham Community Care Special Action Project* Leeds, Nuffield Institute for Health, University of Leeds,

Barr, H (1994) *Perspectives on Shared Learning*, London, UK Centre for the Advancement of Interprofessional Education

Bauman, Z (1992) *Intimations of Postmodernity* London, Routledge

Beck, U (1992) *Risk Society Towards a New Modernity* London, Sage

Beresford, P and Trevillion, S (1995) *Developing Skills for Community Care: a collaborative approach* Aldershot, Arena

Berger, P and Luckman, T (1966) *The Social Construction of Reality A Treatise in the Sociology of Knowledge* London, Penguin

Berkowitz, N (1992) 'Care Management, an American Perspective' in Ramon, S (ed) *Care Management – Implications for Training* Sheffield University Print Unit, ATSWE

Bicstek, F (1961) *The Casework Relationship* London, George Allen & Unwin

Blaug, R (1995) 'Distortion of the face to face: communicative reason and social work practice' *British Journal of Social Work* 25, pp. 423–39

Bornat, J (1997) *Representations of Community' in Community Care: a Reader* (eds) Bornat, J, Johnson, J, Pereira, C, Pilgrim, D and Williams, F London, Macmillan

Boud, D and Knights, S (1996) 'Course design for reflective practice' in *Reflective Learning for Social Work: Research, Theory and Practice* (eds) Gould, N and Taylor, I Aldershot, Arena

Bradley, G and Manthorpe, J (1997) *Dilemmas of Financial Assessment: a practitioner's guide* Birmingham, Venture Press

Bramley, P and Pahl, J (1996) *The Evaluation of Training in the Social Services* London, National Institute for Social Work Research Unit,

Brandon, A (1998) 'Mandy' in Brandon, D and Hawkes, A (eds) *Speaking Truth to Power: Care Planning with Disabled People* Birmingham, Venture Press

Brandon, A and Brandon, D (1987) *Consumers as Colleagues* London, MIND

Brandon, D (1992) 'Skills for service brokerage' in Ramon, S (ed.)*Care Management – Implications for Training* Sheffield University Print Unit, ATSWE

Brandon,D and Brandon,T (2002) *Advocacy in Social Work* Birmingham, Venture Press

Brandon, D and Hawkes, A (1998) *Speaking Truth to Power: care planning with disabled people* Birmingham, Venture Press

Braye, S and Preston-Shoot, M (1995) *Empowering Practice in Social Care* Buckingham, Open University Press

Bright, A and Drake, M (1999) *People with Learning Difficulties and their Access to Direct Payment Schemes* York, Joseph Rowntree Foundation,

Burke, B and Harrison, P (1998) 'Anti-oppressive practice' in Adams, R, Dominelli, L and Payne, M (eds) *Social Work: Themes, Issues and Critical Debates* London, Macmillan

Camilleri, P (1996) *(Re)Constructing Social Work* Aldershot, Avebury

CCETSW (1998) R*eview of the Central Council for Education and Training in Social Work Consultation Documents on Qualifying Education and Training and Post Qualifying Education and Training* London, CCETSW,

Challis, D and Davies, B (1986) *Case Management in Community Care* Aldershot, Gower

Chand, A, Fishwick, C, and Gorman, H, (2001) *Learning Social Care Law* Birmingham, Pepar Publications

Clark, H and Spafford, J (2001) *Piloting Choice and Control for Older People: an Evaluation,*York, Joseph Rowntree Foundation,

Clark, H, Dyer, S and Horwood, J (1998) *'That Bit of Help': the high value of low level preventative services for older people* Bristol, Policy Press/JRF

Clarke, J (1993) 'The comfort of strangers: social work in context' in Clarke, J (ed) *A Crisis in Care: Challenges to Social Work* London, Sage

Clarke, J (1998) 'Thriving on Chaos? Managerialism and Social Welfare' in Carter, J (ed) *Postmodernity and the Fragmentation of Welfare* London, Routledge

Clarke, J and Newman, J (1997) *The Managerial State* London, Sage

Clough, R (1990) *Practice, Politics and Power in Social Services Departments* Aldershot, Avebury

Covey, S (1993) *Principle-Centred Leadership* London, Simon & Schuster

Cree, V (1995) *From Public Streets to Private Lives* Aldershot, Avebury

Croft, S and Beresford, P (2000) 'Empowerment' in Davies, M (ed) *Blackwell Encyclopaedia of Social Work* Oxford, Blackwell

Dant, T and Gearing, B (1990) 'Key workers for elderly people in the community: case managers and care coordinators' *Journal Of Social Policy* 19, pp. 331–60

Dant, T and Gearing, B (1993) 'Key workers for elderly people in the community' in Bornat, J, Pereira, C, Pilgrim, D and Williams, F (eds) *Community Care a Reader*

Davies, C (1983) 'Professions in bureaucracies: the conflict thesis revisited' in Dingwall, R and Lewis, P (eds) *The Sociology of Professions* London, Macmillan

Dawson, C (2000) *Implementing Direct Payments* York, Joseph Rowntree Foundation,

Denzin, N and Lincoln, Y (eds) (1994) *Handbook of Qualitative Research* Thousand Oaks, Sage

Dissenbacher, H (1989) 'Neglect, abuse and the taking of life in old people's Homes' *Ageing and Society* 9, pp 67–71

DOH (Department of Health) (1989) *Caring for People – Community Care in the Next Decade and Beyond Implementation Documents Draft Guidance: assessment and case management* London, Published, HMSO,

DOH (Department of Health) (1990) *Community Care in the Next Decade and Beyond* London, HMSO

DOH (Department of Health) (1997) *The New NHS: modern, dependable* London, HMSO,

DOH (Department of Health) (1998a) *Modernising Health and Social Services: national priorities guidance 1999/00-2001/02* London, HMSO

DOH (Department of Health) (1998b) *Modernising Social Services: promoting independence, improving protection, raising standards* London, HMSO

DOH (Department of Health) (1998c) *National Service Frameworks* HSC (98) 74, London, HMSO

DOH (Department of Health) (1998d) *Partnership in Action: new opportunities for joint working between health and social services: a discussion document* London, HMSO

DOH (Department of Health) (1999) *Social services performance in 1989-99* the personal social services performance assessment framework, London

DOH (Department of Health) (2000a) *The NHS Plan: the Government's response to the Royal Commission on long term care* London

DOH (Department of Health)(2000b) *A Quality Strategy for Social Care* London, HMSO

DOH (Department of Health)(2001) *Developments in Statistical Collections* website: http://wwwdohgovuk/raphtm accessed 14 July 2001

DOH (Department of Health)and Challis, D (1994) *Implementing Caring for People: case management factors influencing its development in the implementation of community care* London, HMSO

DOH/SSI (Department of Health/Social Services Inspectorate (1997) Preparing to Care: Inspection of Social Services Department Planning and Review Processes Relating to the Training Support Programme, London, HMSO,

DOH/SSI (Department of Health/Social Services Inspectorate (1998) *Case Management Study Report on National Data and Care Management Arrangements* London, HMSO

DOH/SSI (Department of Health/Social Services Inspectorate (1999) *Modern Social Services – A Commitment to Improve: The 8th Annual Report of the Chief Inspector of Social Services 1998/1999* website: http://www.dohgovuk/pub/docs/doh/mssactipdf accessed 14 July 2001

Dowson, S (1995) *Increasing User Control in Social Services: the value of the service brokerage model* York, Joseph Rowntree Foundation,

Doyal, L and Gough, I (1991) *A Theory of Human Need* London, Macmillan

England, H (1986) *Social Work as Art* London, Allen & Unwin

England, H (1998) *Social Work as a Profession: the naïve aspiration* 8th Annual CEDR Public Lecture, 15 May 1997 Southampton, CEDR, Department of Social Work Studies, University of Southampton

Eraut, M (1994) *Developing Professional Knowledge and Competence* London, Falmer Press

Fawcett, B (1998) 'Disability and social work: applications from post-structuralism, postmodernism and feminism' *British Journal of Social Work* 28,pp 263–77

Fawcett, B and Featherstone, B (1998) 'Quality Assurance and Evaluation in Social Work in a Postmodern Era' in Carter, J (ed) *Postmodernity and the Fragmentation of Welfare* London, Routledge

Fineman, S (Ed) (1993) *Emotion in Organisations* London, Sage

Fisher, M (1997) 'Research, Knowledge and Practice in Community Care' *Issues in Social Work Education* 17, (2) pp 17–30

Foucault, M (1984) 'Truth and power (from: power/knowledge)' in (ed) Rabinow, P *The Foucault Reader: an introduction to Foucault's thought* London, Penguin

Fox, N (1995) 'Postmodern Perspectives on Care: the vigil and the gift' *Critical Social Policy* 15, pp 107–25

Futter, C and Penhale, B (1996) 'Needs-led Assessment The Practitioner's Perspective' in (eds) Phillips, J and Penhale, B *Reviewing Care Management for Older People* London, Jessica Kingsley

Gaster, L (1995) *Quality in Public Services Managers' Choices* Buckingham, Open University Press

Giddens, A (1991) *Modernity and Self-Identity Self and Society in the Late Modern Age* Cambridge, Polity Press

Giddens, A (1994) *Beyond Left and Right: the Future of Radical Politics* Oxford, Policy Press

Ginsburg, N (1998) 'Postmodernity and Social Europe' in (ed) Carter, J *Postmodernity and the Fragmentation of Welfare* London, Routledge

Glaser, B and Strauss, A (1967) *The Discovery of Grounded Theory* London, Weidenfeld & Nicholson

Gorman, H (1994) *An Exploratory Study of Interest in Postqualification Courses in Community Care* Birmingham, UCE, summarised in Social Services Abstracts (1994) and in CAIPE Bulletin No.7 1994

Gorman, H (1995) 'Learning from experience' *LBTC conference on Training Professionals in Health and Social Care* summarised in CAIPE Bulletin No 9 Summer 1995,pp 23–24

Gorman, H (1996a) 'Reflection on the collaborative process' *Satisfying the Consumer: quality across the boundaries of care* Association for Quality in Healthcare Annual Conference Edgbaston, Birmingham, 22–23 October 1996

Gorman, H (1999a) 'Practitioner Research in Community Care: Personalising the Political' in (ed) Broad, B, *The Politics of Social Work Research and Evaluation* Birmingham, Venture Press ch 12 pp 171–83

Gorman, H (1999b) *Skills, Knowledge and Continuing Education for*

Complex Care Management: a critical evaluation of the roles, tasks and skills of care managers in a context of changing professional identities and the commodification of welfare Unpublished PhD thesis, Faculty of Education, University of Central England in Birmingham

Gorman, H (2000a) 'Collaboration in Community Care and Primary Care' in (ed) Davies, M *The Blackwell Encyclopaedia of Social Work* Oxford, Blackwell pp 67–9

Gorman, H (2000b) 'Winning Hearts and Minds? – Emotional Labour and Learning for Care Management Work' *Journal of Social Work Practice* 14, (2) pp 149–58

Gorman,H (2000c)' The evaluation of planned care: an extra burden for care managers or an opportunity to add value?' *Managing Community Care* 8 (3),pp 20–3

Gorman, H, Gurney, A, Harvey, A, Hutchinson, O, Sylvester, V and Warburton, J (1996) 'The value of analysing the interlocking nature of oppression for those involved in working and learning together in community care' *Journal of Interprofessional Care* 10, (2) pp 147–57

Goss, S and Miller, C (1995) *From Margin to Mainstream – Developing User and Carer Centred Community Care* York, Joseph Rowntree Foundation,

Griffiths, Sir R (1988) *Community Care: agenda for action A report to the Secretary of State for Social Services* London, HMSO

Guba, E and Lincoln, Y (1989) *Fourth Generation Evaluation* Newbury Park, CA, Sage

Hadley, R and Clough, R (1996) *Care in Chaos Frustration and Challenge in Community Care* London, Cassell

Harden, I (1992) *The Contracting State* Buckingham, Open University Press

Harding, T (1997) *A Life Worth Living: The independence and inclusion of older people* London, Help the Aged

Harrison S and Pollit,C, (1994) *Controlling Health Professionals: the future of work and organisation in the NHS* Buckingham, Open University Press

Harvey, D (1989) *The Condition of Postmodernity: an enquiry into the origins of social change* Oxford, Blackwell

Harvey, L, Moon, S, Geall, V and Bowker, R (1997) *Graduates' Work: organisational change and students Attributes* Birmingham, The University of Central England in Birmingham, URC and the Association of Graduate Recruiters,

Hasler, F, Campbell, J and Zarb, G (1999) *Direct Routes to Independence: a huide to local authority implementation and management of direct payments* London, Policy Studies Institute,

Henwood, M (1992) *Through a Glass Darkly Community Care and Elderly People* London, Kings Fund Institute,

Henwood, M (1995) *Making a Difference? Implementation of the Community Care Reforms Two Years On* London, Nuffield Institute for Health, Kings Fund Centre,

Hirst, J (1995) 'Learning to Survive' *Community Care*, 7 December pp 26–7

Hochschild, A (1983) *The Managed Heart: commercialisation of human feeling* Berkley, University of California Press

Holman, B (1993) *A New Deal for Social Welfare* Oxford, Lion Publishing

Holman, B (1998) *Faith in the Poor*, Oxford, Lion Publishing

Holman, B (2000) *Kids at the Door Revisited* Lyme Regis, RHP

Howe, D (1986) *Social Workers and their Practice in Welfare Bureaucracies* Aldershot, Gower

Howe, D (1994) 'Modernity, postmodernity and social work' *British Journal of Social Work* 24, (5) pp 513–32

Howe, D (1996) 'Surface and depth in social work practice' in (ed) Parton, N *Social Theory, Social Change and Social Work* London, Routledge

Hoyes, L, Lart, R, Means, R and Taylor, M (1994) *Community Care in Transition* York, Joseph Rowntree Foundation,

Hudson, B (1993) *The Busy Person's Guide to Care Management* Sheffield, Social Services Monographs Research in Practice

Hughes, B (1995) *Older People and Community Care – Critical Theory and Practice* Buckingham, Open University Press

Hugman, R (1991a) 'Organisation and professionalism: the social work agenda in the 1990s' *British Journal of Social Work* 21, pp 199–216

Hugman, R (1991b) *Power in Caring Professions* London, Macmillan

Hugman, R (1994) 'Social work and case management in the UK: models of professionalism and elderly people' *Ageing and Society* 14, (2) pp 237–53

Humphries, B (1996) 'Contradictions in the culture of empowerment' in (ed) Humphries, B, *Critical Perspecives on Empowerment* Birmingham, Venture Press

Huxley, P (1993) 'Case management and care management in community care' *British Journal of Social Work* 23, pp 365–81

Hyland, T (1994) *Competence, Education and NVQs: dissenting perspectives* London, Cassell

Johnson, T (1972) *Professions and Power* London, Macmillan

Jones, C (1998) 'Social Work and Society' in (eds) Adams, R, Dominelli, L and Payne, M *Social Work: Themes, Issues and Critical Debates* London, Macmillan

Jordan, B (1997) 'Social Work and Society' in (ed) Davies, M *The Blackwell Companion to Social Work* Oxford, Blackwell

Jordan, B (2000) 'Conclusion: tough love: social work practice in UK society' in (eds) Stepney, P and Ford, D *Social Work Models, Methods and Theories: A framework for practice* Lyme Regis, RHP

Jordan, B and Jordan, C (2000) *Social Work and the Third Way: tough love as social policy* London, Sage

Kelly, A (1998) 'Concepts of Professions and Professionalism' in (eds) Symonds, A and Kelly, A *The Social Construction of Community Care* London, Macmillan

Kuhn, T (1962) T*he Structure of Scientific Revolutions* Chicago, University of Chicago Press

Langan, M (1998) 'Radical social work' in (eds) Adams, R, Dominelli, L and Payne, M *Social Work: themes, issues and critical debates* London, Macmillan

Lash, S and Urry, J (1994) *Economics of Signs and Space*, London, Sage

Lass, F (2001) 'Today's choices: Life of Grime Special: Mr Trebus' *Radio Times* 28 April – 4 May 2001, p 104

Le Grand, J and Bartlett, W (1993) *Quasi-Markets and Social Policy* London, Macmillan

Leonard, P (1997) *Postmodern Welfare: reconstructing an emancipatory project* London, Sage

Levick, P (1991) 'The Janus face of community care legislation: an opportunity for radical possibilities' *Critical Social Policy*, 29, pp 75–92

Lewis, H and Milne, A (2000)T*aking Prevention Forward: a directory of examples* website: http://wwwpreventionworksorguk/publications/reportshtm accessed 14 July 2001

Lewis, H, Hardy, B, Waddington, E, Fletcher, P and Milne, A (1999) *Developing a Preventative Approach with Older People* York, Joseph Rowntree Foundation,

Lewis, J and Glennester, H (1996) *Implementing the New Community Care* Buckingham, Open University Press

Lewis, J, Bernstock, P, Bovell, V and Wookey, F (1997) 'Implementing care management: issues in relation to the new community care' *British Journal of Social Work* 27,pp 5–24

Lewis, J, Bernstock, S and Bovell, V (1995) 'The community care changes: unresolved tensions in policy and issues in implementation' *Journal of Social Policy* 24, (1) pp 73–94

Lincoln, Y and Guba, E (1985) *Naturalistic Enquiry* Beverley Hills, CA, Sage

Lipsky, M (1980) Street Level Bureaucracy Dilemmas of the Individual in Public Service, New York, Russel Sage Foundation

Loader, B (1998) 'Welfare direct: informatics and the emergence of self-service welfare?' in (ed) Carter, J *Postmodernity and the Fragmentation of Welfare* London, Routledge

Lymbery, M (1999) 'Lessons for the Past — Learning for the Future: Social Work in Primary Health Care' *European Association of Schools of Social Work: European Social Work: Building Expertise for the 21st Century* Helsinki, June 10–13

Mandelstam, M and Scwehr, B (1995) *Community Care Practice and the Law* London, Macmillan

Marshall, M (1989) 'The sound of silence: who cares about the quality of social work with older people?' in (eds) Rojec, C, Peacock, G and Collins, S *The Haunt of Misery: Critical Essays in Social Work and Helping* London, Routledge

Mayo, M (1994) *Communities and Caring The Mixed Economy of Welfare* London, Macmillan

McLeod, E and Bywaters, P (2000) *Social Work, Health and Equality* London, Routledge

Means, R and Smith, R (1998) *Community Care Policy and Practice* London, Macmillan

Morris, J (1991) *Pride Against Prejudice* London, Women's Press

Mullaly, R (1993) *Structural Social Work: ideology, theory and practice* Toronto, McClelland and Stewart

Nocon, A and Quereshi, H (1996) *Outcomes of Community Care for Users and Carers* Buckingham, Open University Press

Oakland, J (1989) *Total Quality Management* London, Butterworth/Heinemann

O'Brien, M and Penna, S (1998) 'Oppositional postmodern theory and welfare analysis: anti-oppressive practice in a postmodern frame' in (ed) Carter, J *Postmodernity and the Fragmentation of Welfare* London, Routledge

Oliver, M (1990) *The Politics of Disablement* London, Macmillan

Oliver, M (1996) *Understanding Disablitiy: From theory to practice* London, Macmillan

Øÿvretveit, J (1993) *Coordinating Community Care, Multidisciplinary Teams and Care Management* Buckingham, Open University Press

Parton, N (1994) 'Problematics of Government (Post)Modernity and Social Work' *British Journal of Social Work* 24, (1)pp 9–32

Parton, N (Ed) (1996a) *Social Theory, Social Change and Social Work* London, Routledge

Parton, N (1996b) 'Social work, risk and the blaming system' in (ed) Parton, N *Social Theory, Social Change and Social Work* London, Routledge

Payne, M (1995) *Social Work and Community Care* London, Macmillan

Payne, M (1996) *What is Professional Social Work?* Birmingham, Venture Press

Payne, M (1997) 'Care Management and Social Work' in (eds) Bornat, J, Johnson, J, Pereira, C, Pilgrim, D and Williams, F *Community Care: a Reader* London, Macmillan

Payne, M (1998) 'Social work theories and reflective practice' in (eds) Adams, R, Dominelli, L and Payne, M *Social Work: themes, issues and critical debates* London, Macmillan

Payne, M (2000) *Teamwork in Multiprofessional Care* London, Macmillan

Pearson, G (1982) *The Barclay Report and Community Social Work: Samuel Smiles Revisited?* Sheffield Polytechnic, Occassional Paper, Sheffield

Pease, B and Fook, J (1999) 'Postmodern critical theory and emancipatory social work practice' in (eds) Pease, B and Fook, J *Transforming Social Work Practice: Postmodern Critical Perspectives* London, Routledge

Phillips, J (1996) The future of social work with older people in a changing world, in (ed) Parton, N *Social Theory, Social Change and Social Work* London, Routledge

Pilling, D (1992) *Approaches to Care Management for People with Disabilities* London, Jessica Kingsley

Pirsig, R (1974) *Zen and the Art of Motorcycle Maintenance An Inquiry into Values* London, Vintage Books

Pithouse, A (1987) *Social Work: the social organisation of an invisible trade* Aldershot, Avebury

Popple, K (1995) *Analysing Community Work: its theory and practice* Buckingham, Open University Press

Postle, K (1999) *Care Managers' Responses to Working Under Conditions of Postmodernity* Unpublished PhD thesis, Department of Social Work Studies, University of Southampton

Postle, K (2001) 'The social work side is disappearing It started with us being called care managers' *Practice* 13, (1) pp 13–26

Postle, K (2002), 'Working "between the idea and the reality" – ambiguities and tensions in care managers' work' *British Journal of Social Work*, 32, pp 335–51

Postle, K and Ford, P (2000) 'Using mediation skills in family work' in (ed) Wheal, A *Working with Parents: learning from other people's experience* Lyme Regis, Russell House

Power, M (1997) *The Audit Society Rituals of Verification* Oxford, Oxford University Press

Rachman, R (1995) 'Community care: changing the role of hospital social work' *Health and Social Care in the Community*, 3, pp 163–72

Satyamurti, C (1981) *Occupational Survival* Oxford, Blackwell

Schön, D (1987) *Educating the Reflective Practitioner: How Professionals Think in Action* New York, Basic Books

Schön, D (1991) *The Reflective Practitioner how professionals think in action* New York, Basic Books

Schön, D (1992) 'The crisis of professional knowledge and the pursuit of an epistemology of practice' *Journal of Interprofessional Care* 6, (1) pp 49–63

Schorr, A (1992) *The Personal Social Services: an outside view*, York, Joseph Rowntree Foundation

Schwehr, B (1999) *Local Authority Rationing in the Provision of Services* London, Public Law Group: Rowe and Maw Solicitors

Seebohm Report (1968) *Committee on Local Authority and Allied Personal Social Services* London, HMSO,

Servian, R (1996) *Theorising Empowerment: Individual Power and Community Care* Bristol, Policy Press

Shakespeare, T (2000) *Help* Birmingham, Venture Press

Shardlow, S (1999) 'Professional values in social work: the value of 'partnership' ' *European Social Work: Building Expertise for the 21st Century* Helsinki, 10-13 June

Shardlow, S (2000) 'Partnership with Service Users' (ed) Davies, M in *Blackwell Encyclopaedia of Social Work* Oxford, Blackwell

Sheldon, B (1986) 'Social work effectiveness experiments: review and implications' *British Journal of Social Work* 16, pp 223–42

Sheppard, M (1995) *Care Management and the New Social Work: a critical analysis* London, Whiting and Birch

Simiç, P (1995) 'What's in a word? from social "worker" to care "manager"' *Practice* 7, (3) pp 5–18

Simiç, P (1997) 'Social work, primary care and organisational and professional change' *Research, Policy and Planning* 15, (1) pp 1–7

Smale, G and Tuson, G (1992) *Managing Change Through Innovation* London, NISW

Smale, G, Tuson, G, with Biehal, N and Marsh, P (1993) *Empowerment, Assessment, Care Management and the Skilled Worker* London, HMSO

Smale, G, Tuson, G and Statham, D (2000) *Social Work and Social Problems: working towards social inclusion and social change* London, Macmillan

Smart, B (1993) *Postmodernity* London, Routledge

Smith, C, Preston-Shoot, M and Buckley, J (1995) *Community Care Reforms: the views of users and carers* Manchester, Applied Research and Consultancy Centre, University of Manchester,

Specht, H and Courteney, M (1994) *Unfaithful Angels How Social Work has Abandoned its Mission*, New York, Free Press

SSI and SWSG (Social Services Inspectorate/Social work Services Group) (1991a) *Care Management and Assessment – Practitioners' Guide* London, HMSO

SSI and SWSG (Social Services Inspectorate/Social Work Services Group) (1991b) *Care Management and Assessment – Summary of Practice Guidance* London, HMSO

SSI and SWSG (Social Services Inspectorate/Social Work Services Group) (1991c) *Care Management and Assessment Managers' Guide* London, HMSO

Stevenson, O (1995) 'Case Management Does Social Work Have a Future?' *Issues in Social Work Education* 15, (1) pp 48–59

Stevenson, O and Parsloe, P (1993) *Community Care and Empowerment* York, Joseph Rowntree Foundation

Stewart, J and Walsh, K (1992) 'Change in the Management of Public Services' *Public Administration* 70, (4) pp 499–518

Swieringa, J and Wierdsma, A (1992) *Becoming a Learning Organisation Beyond the Learning Curve* Cambridge, Addison-Wesley University Press

Syrett, V, Jones, M and Sercombe, N (1997) 'Implementing Community Care: the congruence of manager and practitioner cultures' *Social Work and Social Sciences Review*, 7, (3) pp 154–69

Townsend, P and Gebhardt, J (1990) *Commit to Quality, New York* John Wiley

Trevillion, S (1993) *Caring in the Community: a Networking Approach to Community Partnership* London, Longman

Ungerson, C (1993) 'Payment for Caring - Mapping a Territory' in (eds) Deakin, N and Page, R *The Costs of Welfare* Aldershot, Avebury

Unity Sale, A (2001) *Caught in the Act?* website: http://<u>wwwcommunity-carecouk/cc_archive/archivedetailsasp?ID=31524</u>, accessed 13 July

Valios, N (2001) Wheeling-dealing therapies, *Community Care* 7 June pp 30–1

Walsh, L and Woodward, P (1989) 'Continuing professional development: towards a national strategy report for FE Department of DES' in (eds) Watkins, L, Drury, L and Preddy, D *From Evolution to Revolution The Pressures on Professional Life in the 1990s* Bristol, University of Bristol

Webb, S, Moriarty, J and Levin, E (1998) 'Research on community care: social work and community care & community care arrangements for older people with dementia' London, NISW,

Wilson, G (Ed) (1995) *Community Care Asking the Users* London, Chapman and Hall

Wistow, G, Knapp, M Hardy, B Allen, C (1994) *Social Care in a Mixed Economy* Buckingham, Open University Press

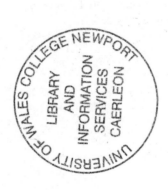